# Electrocardiography:

## Essentials of Interpretation

# Electrocardiography:
## Essentials of Interpretation

**NORA GOLDSCHLAGER, MD**

Clinical Professor of Medicine
University of California School of Medicine
San Francisco

**MERVIN J. GOLDMAN, MD**

Clinical Professor of Medicine
University of California School of Medicine
San Francisco

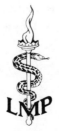

**LANGE Medical Publications**    Los Altos, California 94022

International Standard Book Number: *0-87041-290-6*
Library of Congress Catalogue Card Number: *84-81105*

Electrocardiography: Essentials of Interpretation

A Concise Medical Library for Practitioner and Student

| | |
|---|---|
| **Current Medical Diagnosis & Treatment 1984** (annual revision). Edited by M.A. Krupp and M.J. Chatton. 1153 pp. | 1984 |
| **Current Pediatric Diagnosis & Treatment,** 8th ed. Edited by C.H. Kempe, H.K. Silver, and D. O'Brien. 1164 pp, *illus.* | 1984 |
| **Current Surgical Diagnosis & Treatment,** 6th ed. Edited by L.W. Way. 1221 pp, *illus.* | 1983 |
| **Current Obstetric & Gynecologic Diagnosis & Treatment,** 4th ed. Edited by R.C. Benson. 1038 pp, *illus.* | 1982 |
| **Current Emergency Diagnosis & Treatment.** Edited by J. Mills, M.T. Ho, and D.D. Trunkey. 738 pp, *illus.* | 1983 |
| **Harper's Review of Biochemistry** (formerly **Review of Physiological Chemistry**), 19th ed. D.W. Martin, Jr., P.A. Mayes, and V.W. Rodwell. 638 pp, *illus.* | 1983 |
| **Review of Medical Physiology,** 11th ed. W.F. Ganong. 643 pp, *illus.* | 1983 |
| **Review of Medical Microbiology,** 16th ed. E. Jawetz, J.L. Melnick, and E.A. Adelberg. 557 pp, *illus.* | 1984 |
| **Basic & Clinical Endocrinology.** Edited by F.S. Greenspan and P.H. Forsham. 646 pp, *illus.* | 1983 |
| **Basic & Clinical Pharmacology,** 2nd ed. Edited by B.G. Katzung. 888 pp, *illus.* | 1984 |
| **Basic & Clinical Immunology,** 5th ed. Edited by D.P. Stites, J.D. Stobo, H.H. Fudenberg, and J.V. Wells. About 800 pp, *illus.* | 1984 |
| **Basic Histology,** 4th ed. L.C. Junqueira and J. Carneiro. 510 pp, *illus.* | 1983 |
| **Clinical Cardiology,** 3rd ed. M. Sokolow and M.B. McIlroy. 763 pp, *illus.* | 1981 |
| **General Urology,** 10th ed. D.R. Smith. 598 pp, *illus.* | 1981 |
| **General Ophthalmology,** 10th ed. D. Vaughan and T. Asbury. 407 pp, *illus.* | 1983 |
| **Correlative Neuroanatomy & Functional Neurology,** 18th ed. J.G. Chusid. 476 pp, *illus.* | 1982 |
| **Principles of Clinical Electrocardiography,** 11th ed. M.J. Goldman. 438 pp, *illus.* | 1982 |
| **Handbook of Obstetrics & Gynecology,** 8th ed. R.C. Benson. 804 pp, *illus.* | 1983 |
| **Physician's Handbook,** 20th ed. M.A. Krupp, L.M. Tierney, Jr., E. Jawetz, R.L. Roe, and C.A. Camargo. 774 pp, *illus.* | 1982 |
| **Handbook of Pediatrics,** 14th ed. H.K. Silver, C.H. Kempe, and H.B. Bruyn. 883 pp, *illus.* | 1983 |
| **Handbook of Poisoning: Prevention, Diagnosis, & Treatment,** 11th ed. R.H. Dreisbach. 632 pp. | 1983 |

# Table of Contents

# Preface

Recent advances in electrophysiology have helped to clarify both basic and complex mechanisms of normal and abnormal conduction of the cardiac impulse and the production, maintenance, and termination of arrhythmias. This new body of knowledge has immediate relevance for clinical electrocardiography, since better explanations can now be offered of certain electrocardiographic patterns. Similarly, newer developments in the fields of nuclear cardiology, echocardiography, and angiography have helped to validate some concepts in clinical electrocardiography while invalidating others.

Accordingly, a new introductory book on the essentials of interpretation of clinical electrocardiograms was thought to be both timely and necessary. This book is aimed at students who seek a firm ground upon which to build their understanding of electrocardiographic interpretation. Most important is correlation of the information presented here with the specific clinical setting of which the electrocardiogram is one part, since only by clinical correlation is a diagnostic tool such as the electrocardiogram properly interpreted.

*Principles of Clinical Electrocardiography,* now in its 11th edition, will continue to be revised and reissued triennially. Comments from readers about both books will be welcomed, since it is the authors' intention to keep pace with advances in this scientific field.

Nora Goldschlager, MD
Mervin J. Goldman, MD

San Francisco
July, 1984

# Introduction to Electrocardiography | 1

The electrocardiogram (ECG) is a graphic recording of the electrical potentials produced by cardiac tissue. The heart is unique among the muscles of the body in that it possesses the properties of automatic impulse formation and rhythmic contraction. Electrical impulse formation occurs within the conduction system of the heart; excitation of the muscle fibers throughout the myocardium results in cardiac contraction. Formation and conduction of these electrical impulses produce weak electrical currents that spread through the body. The ECG is recorded by applying electrodes to various locations on the body surface and connecting them to a recording apparatus. The connections of the apparatus are such that an upright deflection indicates positive potential and a downward deflection negative potential.

The ECG is of diagnostic value in the following clinical circumstances: (1) atrial and ventricular hypertrophy; (2) conduction delay of atrial and ventricular electrical impulses; (3) myocardial ischemia and infarction; (4) determination of the origin and monitoring the behavior of dysrhythmias; (5) pericarditis; (6) systemic diseases that affect the heart; (7) determination of the effect of cardiac drugs, especially digitalis and certain antiarrhythmic agents; (8) disturbances in electrolyte balance, especially potassium; and (9) evaluation of function of cardiac pacemakers.

The ECG is a laboratory test, not a sine qua non of the diagnosis of heart disease. A patient with heart disease may have a normal ECG, and a normal individual may have an abnormal ECG. All too often, a patient is made a cardiac invalid solely on the basis of some abnormality on the ECG; on the other hand, a patient may receive unwarranted assurance of the absence of heart disease solely on the basis of a normal ECG. The ECG must *always* be interpreted in the light of surrounding clinical circumstances.

## BIPOLAR STANDARD LEADS

The bipolar standard leads (I, II, and III) are the original leads selected by Einthoven to record electrical potentials in the frontal plane. Electrodes are applied to the left arm (LA), right arm (RA), and left leg (LL). Proper skin contact must be made by rubbing electrode paste on the skin. The LA, RA, and LL leads are then attached to their respective electrodes. By turning the selector dial of the recording apparatus to 1, 2, and 3, the standard leads (I, II, and III) are recorded (Fig 1–1).

Electrocardiographic machines also have a right leg (RL) electrode and lead, which acts as a ground and plays no role in the production of the ECG. In areas where there is electrical interference, it may be necessary to run a ground wire from the bed or from the machine to an appropriate ground (water pipe or steam pipe).

### Electrical Potentials

The bipolar leads represent a difference of electrical potential between 2 selected sites (Fig 1–2):

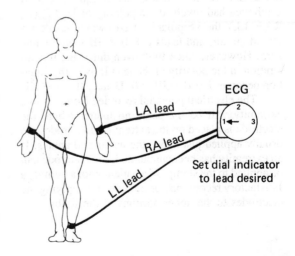

Figure 1–1. Standard leads.

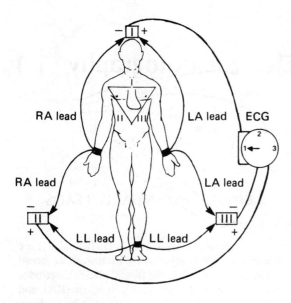

**Figure 1–2.** Connections for bipolar standard leads I, II, and III.

Lead I = Difference of potential between the left arm and the right arm (LA − RA).

Lead II = Difference of potential between the left leg and the right arm (LL − RA).

Lead III = Difference of potential between the left leg and the left arm (LL − LA).

The relation between the 3 leads is expressed algebraically by Einthoven's equation: lead II = lead I + lead III. This is based on Kirchhoff's law, which states that the algebraic sum of all the potential differences in a closed circuit equals zero. If Einthoven had reversed the polarity of lead II (ie, RA − LL), the 3 bipolar lead axes would result in a closed circuit, and leads I + II + III would equal zero. However, since Einthoven did make this alteration in the polarity of the lead II axis, the equation becomes I − II + III = 0. Hence, II = I + III.

The electrical potential recorded from any one extremity will be the same no matter where the electrode is placed on the extremity. Electrodes are usually applied just above the wrists and ankles. If an extremity has been amputated, the electrode can be applied to the stump. In a patient with a tremor, a satisfactory record may be obtained by applying the electrodes to the upper portions of the limbs.

# UNIPOLAR LEADS
## (Extremity Leads, Precordial [Chest] Leads, Esophageal Leads, Intracardiac Leads)

Unipolar leads (VR, VL, and VF), precordial leads (V), and esophageal leads (E) were introduced into clinical electrocardiography by Wilson in 1932; unipolar intracardiac leads were introduced a decade later. The frontal plane unipolar leads (VR, VL, and VF) bear a definite mathematical relation to the standard bipolar leads (I, II, and III). The precordial (V) leads record potentials in the horizontal plane without being influenced by potentials from an "indifferent" electrode. Any unipolar lead records not only the electrical potential from a small area of underlying myocardium but also *all* of the electrical events of the entire cardiac cycle as viewed from that site.

### Augmented Extremity Leads
### aVR, aVL, & aVF (Fig 1–3)

By a technique automatically accomplished by all modern electrocardiographic machines, the amplitude of the deflections of VR, VL, and VF can be increased by about 50%. These leads are called augmented unipolar extremity leads and are designated as aVR, aVL, and aVF. Using lead aVR as an example, this augmentation can be illustrated as follows. Since aVR represents a difference of potential between the right arm (RA or VR) and the average of the potential of the left leg and left arm, equation (1) can be established.

$$\textbf{(1)} \quad \textbf{aVR} = \textbf{RA} - \frac{\textbf{LL} + \textbf{LA}}{\textbf{2}}$$

By changing signs in (1),

$$\textbf{(2)} \quad \textbf{aVR} = \textbf{RA} + \left[ -\frac{\textbf{LL} + \textbf{LA}}{\textbf{2}} \right]$$

From Einthoven's equation it is known that

$$\textbf{(3)} \quad \textbf{RA} + \textbf{LA} + \textbf{LL} = \textbf{0}$$

By subtracting LA + LL from both sides of (3),

$$\textbf{(4)} \quad \textbf{RA} = -\ (\textbf{LA} + \textbf{LL})$$

By substituting equation (4) in (2),

$$\textbf{(5)} \quad \textbf{aVR} = \textbf{RA} + \frac{\textbf{RA}}{\textbf{2}} = \textbf{3/2 RA (or 3/2 VR)}$$

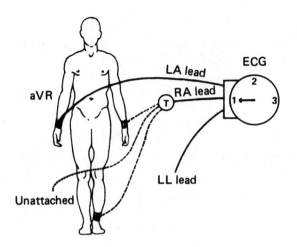

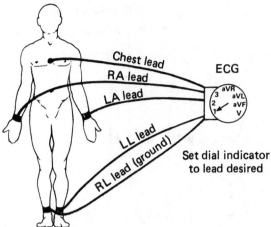

Figure 1–4. Unipolar leads.

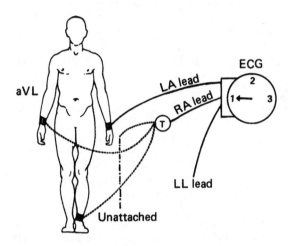

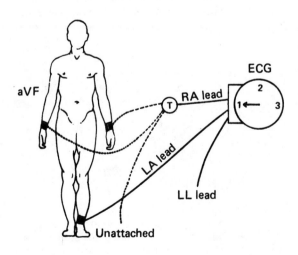

Figure 1–3. Augmented extremity leads.

The only difference between leads VR, VL, and VF and leads aVR, aVL, and aVF is a difference in amplitude. In routine practice, the augmented unipolar extremity leads have replaced the nonaugmented leads because they are easier to read.

Electrocardiographic machines are constructed so that the augmented extremity leads can be recorded using the same hookup as that used for standard leads, by turning the selector dial to aVR, aVL, and aVF. Unipolar precordial leads are recorded by applying the chest lead and electrode to any desired position on the chest and turning the selector dial to the V position (Fig 1–4). Multiple chest leads are recorded by changing the position of the chest electrode. Unipolar esophageal leads are recorded by attaching the esophageal electrode to the chest lead and turning the selector dial to the V position. Unipolar intracardiac leads are recorded by attaching the intracardiac electrode to the chest lead and turning the selector dial to the V position.

## UNIPOLAR PRECORDIAL LEADS

The unipolar precordial leads are obtained by turning the selector dial to V and recording from the various precordial positions. By convention, these precordial positions are as follows (Fig 1–5):

$V_1$: Fourth intercostal space, right sternal border.

$V_2$: Fourth intercostal space, left sternal border.

$V_3$: Equidistant between $V_2$ and $V_4$.

$V_4$: Fifth intercostal space, left midclavicular line. All subsequent leads ($V_{5-9}$) are taken in the same horizontal plane as $V_4$.

$V_5$: Anterior axillary line.

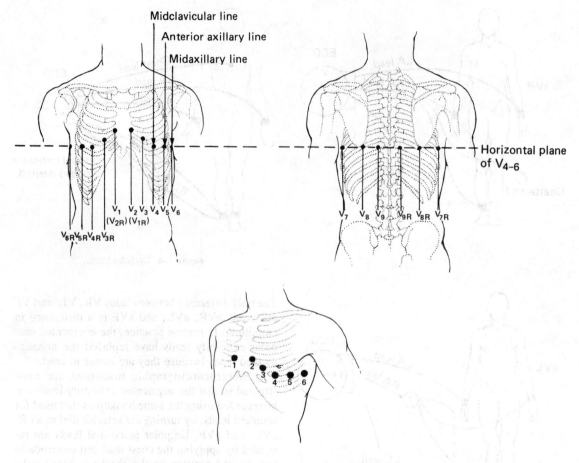

**Figure 1–5.** Locations of the unipolar precordial leads on the body surface.

$V_6$: Midaxillary line.

$V_7$: Posterior axillary line.

$V_8$: Posterior scapular line.

$V_9$: Left border of the spine.

$V_{3R-9R}$: Right side of the chest in the same location as the left-sided leads $V_{3-9}$. $V_{2R}$ is therefore the same as $V_1$.

$3V_{1-9}$: One interspace higher than $V_{1-9}$; these are the third interspace leads. The same terminology can be applied to leads taken in other interspaces, eg, $2V_{1-9}$, $6V_{1-9}$, etc.

The usual routine ECG consists of 12 leads: I, II, III; aVR, aVL, aVF; and $V_{1-6}$.

## MONITOR LEADS

Although it is possible to use any lead (or multiple leads if equipment is available) in a specialized area such as a coronary care unit, it is more common to use a modified bipolar chest lead. The positive electrode is placed in the usual $V_1$ position and the negative electrode near the left shoulder. A third electrode is placed at a more remote area of the chest and serves as a ground (Fig 1–6). The recording will be similar to a modified chest lead ($MCL_1$). This lead is of major value in

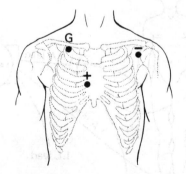

**Figure 1–6.** Modified chest lead (MCL) system for monitoring. The positive electrode is placed in the $V_1$ position, the negative electrode near the left shoulder, and the ground electrode at a remote area of the chest. By changing the placement of the positive electrode, any MCL lead may be recorded.

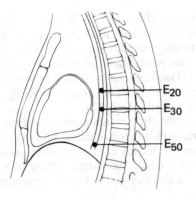

**Figure 1–7.** Sagittal view of the thorax illustrating positions of esophageal electrodes.

rhythm evaluation. However, if it is deemed necessary to monitor the patient for ST–T changes due to ischemia, it is advisable to place the positive electrode in the $V_4$ or $V_5$ position ($MCL_4$ or $MCL_5$) or in any position that is expected or has been noted to show the abnormality.

## UNIPOLAR ESOPHAGEAL LEADS

Esophageal leads are recorded by attaching an esophageal lead to the V (chest) lead of the machine. An electrode catheter is either swallowed or passed through the nares into the esophagus. Using this as one terminal and the zero potential as the other terminal, a unipolar esophageal ("E") lead can be obtained. The nomenclature of the lead is derived from the distance in centimeters from the tip of the nares to the electrode. Thus, $E_{50}$ represents an esophageal electrode located 50 cm from the nares. Leads $E_{40-50}$ usually record the posterior surface of the left ventricle; leads $E_{15-25}$, the atrial area; and leads $E_{25-35}$, the region of the atrioventricular groove (Fig 1–7). Since these positions vary with individual differences in body size and shape and heart position, interpretation of precise electrode location should not be made from a single esophageal lead; a series of low to high esophageal

lead recordings must be made for proper evaluation. For more accurate localization of the position of the esophageal electrode, fluoroscopy may be used.

Esophageal leads are especially useful in recording atrial complexes, which are greatly magnified at this location, and in exploring the posterior surface of the left ventricle.

## UNIPOLAR INTRACARDIAC LEADS

Unipolar intracardiac recordings (electrograms) are made by attaching an electrode catheter to the V (chest) lead and turning the selector dial to the V position. Unipolar electrograms can be recorded from various intracardiac chambers, depending upon the location of the catheter electrodes. Intracardiac electrography is of great clinical value in the assessment of dysrhythmias by amplification of atrial electrical activity (Fig 1–8) and in the proper positioning of a pacing catheter "floated" into the heart without fluoroscopic guidance. In the latter circumstance, the contour and relative sizes of the atrial and ventricular deflections will help identify the location of the catheter tip.

With appropriate electrode catheters inserted into the heart under fluoroscopic guidance, recordings can be made of bundle of His and proximal portions of the bundle branches. This technique, which is limited to the cardiac laboratory, has resulted in major advances in the understanding and interpretation of dysrhythmias and atrioventricular conduction. Intracardiac recordings from multiple sites during intracardiac electrical stimulation can also be made in special laboratories. These recordings are of value in determining the site of origin of tachycardias and their conduction pathways, elucidating the presence of accessory atrioventricular bypass tracts (see Chapter 16), and inducing clinically significant dysrhythmias so the best form of management can be chosen.

Attachment of the V lead to a pericardiocentesis needle, under sterile precautions, permits electrocardiographic recording during this procedure. When the needle meets the epicardium, ST eleva-

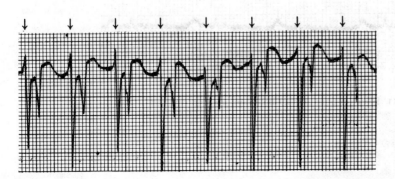

**Figure 1–8.** Unipolar intracardiac electrogram recorded from a catheter electrode positioned in the right atrium. The large, narrow diphasic complexes (arrows) represent atrial activity, and the broad deflections that follow them represent ventricular activity. Simultaneous recording of the intracardiac electrogram and a surface electrocardiographic lead can help to clarify the origin of the intracardiac deflections.

tion will be recorded and is an indication for withdrawing the needle and beginning aspiration.

In all situations in which an electrode is in direct contact with the myocardium, proper electrical grounding is essential. Currents as low as 10 $\mu$A can induce ventricular fibrillation.

## TECHNICAL DIFFICULTIES AFFECTING THE ELECTROCARDIOGRAM

Attention to the following details will ensure against artifacts and poor technical records:

(1) The ECG should be recorded with the patient lying on a comfortable bed or table large enough to support the entire body. The patient must be completely relaxed in order to ensure a satisfactory tracing (Fig 1–9). It is best to explain the procedure in advance to an apprehensive patient in order to allay anxiety. Muscular motions or twitchings by the patient can alter the record (Fig 1–10).

(2) Good contact must exist between the skin and the electrode. Poor contact can result in a suboptimal record (Fig 1–11).

(3) The electrocardiographic machine must be properly standardized so that 1 millivolt (mV) will produce a deflection of 1 cm. Incorrect standardization will produce inaccurate voltage of the complexes, which can lead to faulty interpretation (Fig 1–12).

(4) The patient and the machine must be properly grounded to avoid alternating current interference (Fig 1–13).

(5) Any electronic equipment in contact with the patient, eg, an electrically regulated intravenous infusion pump, can produce artifacts in the ECG (Fig 1–14).

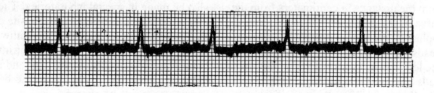

**Figure 1–9.** A technically good tracing.

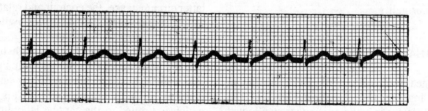

**Figure 1–10.** Effect of muscle twitchings.

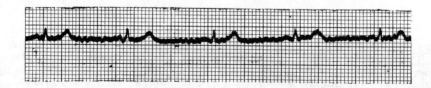

**Figure 1–11.** Effect of poor contact between skin and electrode.

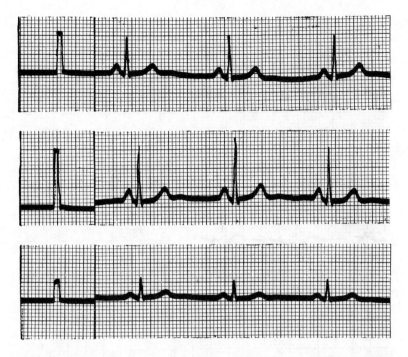

**Figure 1–12.** Effect of standardization. *Top:* Proper standardization: 1-cm deflection. *Middle:* Overstandardization: 1.4-cm deflection. This increases the voltage of the complexes. *Bottom:* Understandardization: 0.5-cm deflection. This decreases the voltage of the complexes.

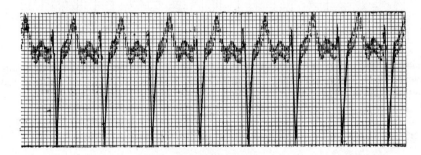

**Figure 1–13.** Effect of alternating current interference.

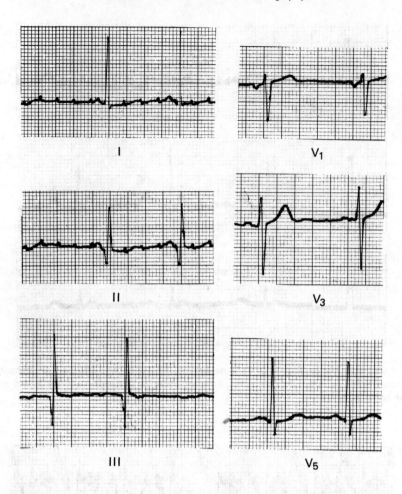

**Figure 1–14.** Regular deflections at a rate of 300/min are recorded in leads I and II, which could result in an interpretation of atrial flutter. However, lead III and the precordial leads indicate sinus rhythm. The deflections occurring at this rapid rate were due to an artifact from an intravenous infusion pump unit inserted into a right forearm vein.

## Intracellular Action Potentials

Four electrophysiologic events are involved in the genesis of the ECG: (1) impulse formation in the primary pacemaker of the heart (usually the sinoatrial node); (2) transmission of the impulse through specialized conduction fibers; (3) activation (depolarization) of the myocardium; and (4) repolarization (recovery) of the myocardium.

If an electrode is placed on the surface of a resting myocardial cell and a second (indifferent) electrode is placed in a remote location, no electrical potential (zero potential) is recorded because of the high impedance of the cell membrane. However, if the cell membrane is penetrated by an electrode, a negative potential of about $-90$ mV will be recorded. This potential is known as the **membrane resting potential** (Fig 2–1). The major factor that determines the resting potential is the gradient of potassium ions ($K^+$) across the cell membrane. The

intracellular concentration of $K^+$ is about 150 meq/L, and the extracellular concentration is about 5 meq/L, resulting in a 30:1 concentration gradient. An opposite gradient exists for sodium ions ($Na^+$), resulting in a high extracellular $Na^+$ concentration relative to intracellular $Na^+$ concentration. The $Na^+$ gradient does not alter the resting potential appreciably, because the cell membrane is considerably less permeable to $Na^+$ than to $K^+$.

At the onset of depolarization of a myocardial cell, there is an abrupt change in permeability of the cell membrane to $Na^+$. $Na^+$ (and, to a lesser extent, calcium ions [$Ca^{2+}$]) enter the cell and result in a sharp rise of intracellular potential to positivity (about $+20$ mV) (Fig 2–1). This phase of depolarization is designated **phase 0** and reflects the $Na^+$-dependent **fast inward current** typical of working myocardial cells and Purkinje fibers. Pacemaker cells in the sinoatrial (SA) and atrioventricular (AV)

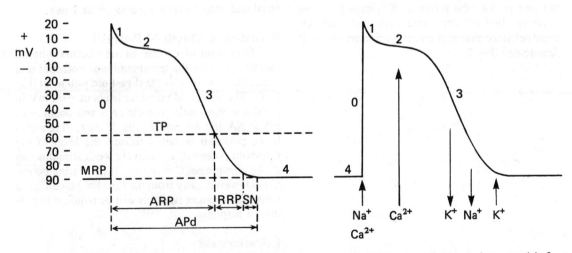

**Figure 2–1.** Diagrams of the action potential of a ventricular muscle cell. MRP = membrane resting potential; 0 = depolarization; 1, 2, 3 = phases of repolarization; 4 = diastolic phase; APd = duration of action potential; TP = threshold potential; ARP = absolute refractory period; RRP = relative refractory period; SN = supernormal period of excitability. Phase 4: Membrane resting potential = $-90$ mV. Phase 0: Rapid depolarization due to $Na^+$ (and $Ca^{2+}$) influx. Phase 1: Initial phase of repolarization. Phase 2: Plateau phase of repolarization in which there is a slow influx of $Ca^{2+}$. Phase 3: Efflux of $K^+$ resulting in slow return of intracellular potential to $-90$ mV. At the termination of phase 3 an active transport system extrudes $Na^+$ from the cell and pumps $K^+$ into the cell.

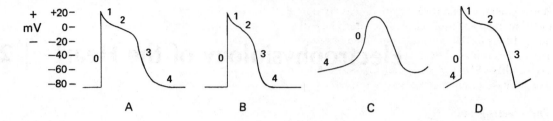

**Figure 2–2.** Diagrams of the action potentials of various cell types within the heart. *A:* Ventricular muscle cell. *B:* Atrial muscle cell. *C:* SA or AV nodal cell. *D:* Purkinje cell. Note the differences between the $Na^+$-dependent working myocardial cells (A and B), whose phase 4 is flat, and the $Ca^{2+}$-dependent cells (C and D) (which have automaticity), whose phase 4 rises toward activation threshold during diastole. This **diastolic depolarization** characterizes automatic cells, as once threshold is spontaneously attained, cellular activation occurs.

nodes are depolarized by a $Ca^{2+}$-dependent **slow inward current.** Under certain abnormal conditions, such as ischemia, cells whose fast inward current of $Na^+$ is inhibited are depolarized by slow inward currents of $Ca^{2+}$.

Following cellular depolarization, there is a gradual return of potential to the resting potential. This **repolarization** process is divided into 3 phases: **phase 1:** an initial rapid return of intracellular potential to 0 mV, largely the result of closing of the $Na^+$ channels; **phase 2:** a plateau resulting from the slow entry of $Ca^{2+}$ into the cell; and **phase 3:** return of the intracellular potential to resting potential, resulting from extrusion of $K^+$ out of the cell. At the end of phase 3, the normal negative resting potential is reestablished; however, the cell is left with an excess of $Na^+$ and a deficit of $K^+$. A $Na^+$-$K^+$ pump, which removes $Na^+$ from the cell and permits the influx of $K^+$, then becomes effective. In $Ca^{2+}$-dependent cells (SA and AV nodal cells) the phases of repolarization are less well demarcated (Fig 2–2).

The summation of all phase 0 potentials of atrial myocardial cells results in the P wave inscribed in the ECG. Phase 2 corresponds to the PR segment, which follows the P wave (see Chapter 3), and phase 3 corresponds to the $T_a$ wave of atrial repolarization. The summation of phase 0 potentials of ventricular myocardial cells results in the QRS complex in the ECG. Phase 2 corresponds to the ST segment and phase 3 to the T wave (Fig 2–3).

**Conduction Velocity**

The speed at which electrical impulses spread through the heart varies considerably and depends upon the intrinsic properties of different portions of the conduction system and myocardium. Conduction velocity is most rapid in the His bundle and Purkinje system (about 2 m/s) and slowest in the SA and AV nodes (0.01–0.02 m/s); conduction within atrial and ventricular muscle is about 1 m/s.

**Excitation & Threshold Potential**

Excitation of cardiac muscle occurs when a stimulus reduces the transmembrane potential to a critical level known as the **threshold potential** (Fig 2–1). The threshold potential is about −60 mV in atrial and ventricular muscle cells and about −40 mV in SA and AV nodal cells. If the resting membrane potential is raised toward the level of the threshold potential, a relatively weak stimulus can evoke a response. Conversely, if the resting potential is lowered away from the threshold potential, a relatively stronger stimulus will be required to produce a response.

**Refractoriness**

The refractory period of myocardial tissue is divided into the **absolute refractory period** (ARP; Fig 2–1), during which no stimulus of any intensity can evoke a response, and a **relative (effective) refractory period** (RRP; Fig 2–1), during which only a strong stimulus can evoke a response. The ARP includes phases 0, 1, 2, and part of 3 of the

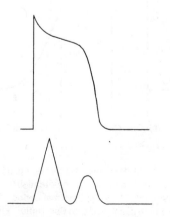

**Figure 2–3.** Diagram of the relation between the action potential of a ventricular myocardial cell and the surface recording of the resulting depolarization and repolarization.

action potential. The RRP begins at about the time the membrane potential reaches the threshold potential and ends just before the termination of phase 3. The RRP is followed by the period of **supernormal excitability** (SN; Fig 2–1), during which a relatively weak stimulus can evoke a response.

## The Electrogram

A recording of the electrical potentials of a stimulated muscle is analogous to a unipolar ECG and is termed an **electrogram.** There are 2 parts to an electrogram: depolarization (the deflection produced during passage of the electrical stimulus through the muscle) and repolarization (the deflection produced during return of the muscle to a resting state) (Fig 2–4). The direction in which a stimulus spreads through the muscle and the position of the recording electrode relative to the direction of spread of the impulse will determine its polarity in the recording (Fig 2–5). If muscles of different masses are stimulated, the electrical potentials recorded will reflect the net depolarization and repolarization (Fig 2–6).

The time required for the spread of the impulse

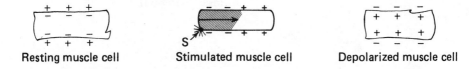

| Resting muscle cell | Stimulated muscle cell | Depolarized muscle cell |

**Figure 2–4.** Diagrams of resting, stimulated, and depolarized muscle cells. When the muscle is stimulated (S = stimulus), the surface of the stimulated portion of the muscle becomes electrically negative. As the impulse traverses the muscle, there is an advancing negative charge. The portion of muscle that has not yet received the stimulus is electrically positive.

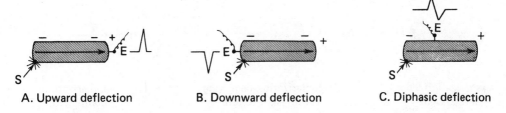

| A. Upward deflection | B. Downward deflection | C. Diphasic deflection |

**Figure 2–5.** Electrical deflections produced by muscle stimulation. *A:* The upward deflection is produced by the spread of the stimulus (S) toward an electrode (E) located at the positively charged end of the muscle. *B:* Downward deflection produced by spread of the impulse away from an electrode located at the negatively charged end of the muscle. *C:* Diphasic deflection, recorded by an electrode positioned at the mid portion of the muscle, produced by the initial advancing positive charge and subsequent passing negative charge.

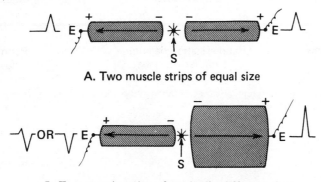

A. Two muscle strips of equal size

B. Two muscle strips of markedly different sizes

**Figure 2–6.** *A:* Muscles of equal size. If 2 muscle strips of approximately equal size are stimulated at a central point, a positive deflection (of depolarization) of equal magnitude will be recorded at both ends. *B:* Muscles of unequal size. If 2 muscle masses of markedly different sizes (analogous to the right and left ventricles) are stimulated at a central point, a large positive deflection will be recorded over the larger muscle mass, and a small positive deflection followed by a deep negative deflection (or an entirely negative deflection) will be recorded over the smaller muscle mass. This negative deflection is due to the fact that the *net* deflection of depolarization is directed away from the smaller muscle mass.

from the stimulated end of a muscle to the opposite end can be measured on the electrogram from the onset of the depolarization deflection to its peak. In clinical electrocardiography, an approximation of this time, measured from the onset of the inscription of the complex to its peak, is termed the **intrinsic (intrinsicoid) deflection** or **activation time**; the measurement is usually applied only to QRS complexes (Fig 2–7).

During repolarization, the muscle returns to its resting state. If repolarization occurs in a direction opposite to that of depolarization, the repolarization deflection will be in the same direction as that produced by the depolarization deflection (Fig 2–8A). If repolarization occurs in the same direction as that of depolarization, the repolarization deflection will be opposite to that of the depolarization deflection (Fig 2–8B).

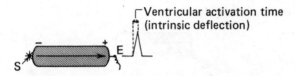

**Figure 2–7.** The intrinsic (intrinsicoid) deflection, or ventricular activation time, is a measure of the time taken by impulse propagation from one end of the stimulated muscle to the other.

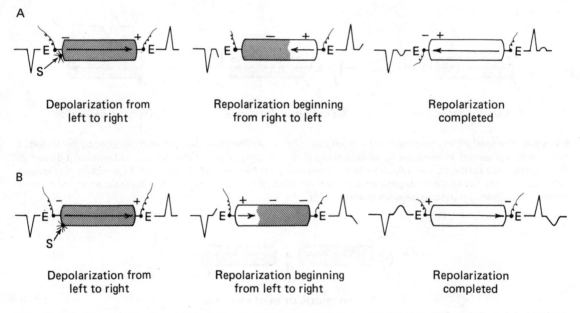

**Figure 2–8.** *A:* Depolarization from left to right and repolarization in the opposite direction. *B:* Depolarization from left to right and repolarization in the same direction.

# Definitions of Electrocardiographic Configurations | 3

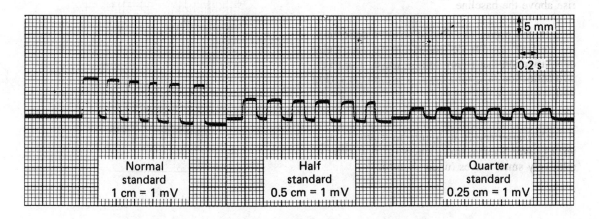

Figure 3–1. Electrocardiographic paper and 1-mV calibration signals.

## The Electrocardiographic Grid

Electrocardiographic paper is graph paper with horizontal and vertical lines at 1-mm intervals. A heavier line is present every 5 mm. Time is measured along the horizontal lines: 1 mm = 0.04 s; 5 mm = 0.2 s (Fig 3–1). Voltage is measured along the vertical lines and is expressed as mm (10 mm = 1 mV). In routine practice, the recording speed is 25 mm/s. The usual calibration is a 1-mV signal that produces a 10-mm deflection. "Double standard" produces a 20-mm deflection, "half standard" produces a 5-mm deflection, and "quarter standard" produces a 2.5-mm deflection (Fig 3–1).

## NORMAL ELECTROCARDIOGRAPHIC COMPLEXES

**P wave:** The deflection produced by atrial depolarization (Fig 3–2).

**$T_a$ wave:** The deflection produced by atrial repolarization. This deflection is usually not seen in the 12-lead ECG (Fig 3–2).

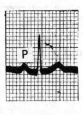

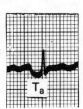

Figure 3–2. The P and $T_a$ waves.

**Q (q) wave:** The initial negative deflection resulting from ventricular depolarization (Fig 3–3).

**R (r) wave:** The first positive deflection resulting from ventricular depolarization (Fig 3–3).

**S (s) wave:** The first negative deflection of ventricular depolarization that follows the first positive deflection (R) (Fig 3–3).

**QS wave:** A negative deflection that does not rise above the baseline.

**R′ (r′) wave:** The second positive deflection, ie, the first positive deflection during ventricular depolarization that follows the S wave. The negative deflection following the r′ is termed the s′ (Fig 3–3).

Capital letters (Q, R, S) refer to relatively large waves (over 5 mm); small letters (q, r, s) refer to relatively small waves (under 5 mm).

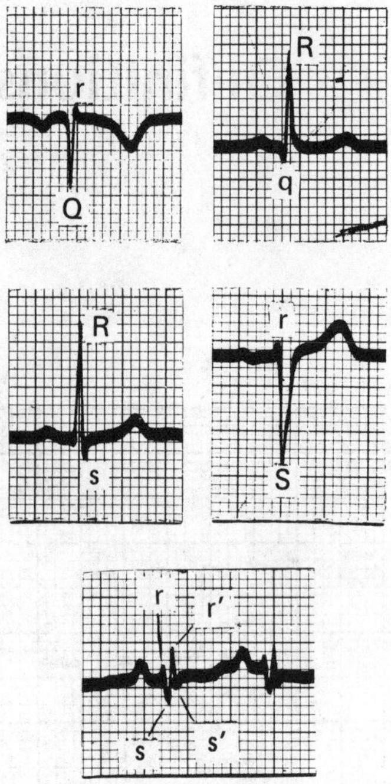

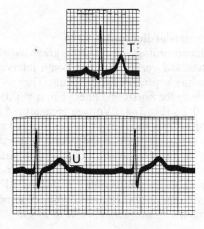

**Figure 3–3.** The QRS complex.

**T wave:** The deflection produced by ventricular repolarization (Fig 3–4).

**U wave:** The deflection (usually positive) seen following the T wave but preceding the next P wave. The cause of this wave is thought to be repolarization of the intraventricular (Purkinje) conduction system (Fig 3–4).

**Figure 3–4.** The T and U waves.

## NORMAL INTERVALS

**RR interval** (Fig 3–5): The RR interval is the distance between 2 successive R waves. If the ventricular rhythm is regular, the interval in seconds (or fractions of a second) between 2 successive R waves divided into 60 (seconds) will give the heart rate per minute. If the ventricular rhythm is irregular, the number of R waves in a given period of time (eg, 10 s) should be counted and the results converted into the number per minute. For example, if 20 R waves are counted in a 10-s interval, the ventricular rate is 120 per minute (20 × 6).

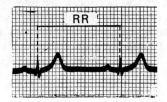

**PP interval** (Fig 3–5): In regular sinus rhythm, the PP interval will be the same as the RR interval. However, when the ventricular rhythm is irregular or when atrial and ventricular rates are regular but different from each other, the PP interval should be measured from the same point on 2 successive P waves and the atrial rate per minute computed in the same manner as the ventricular rate.

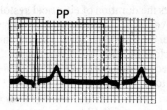

**PR interval** (Fig 3–5): This measures the AV conduction time. It includes the time required for (1) atrial depolarization, (2) the normal conduction delay in the AV node (approximately 0.07 s), and (3) the passage of the impulse through the bundle of His and bundle branches to the onset of ventricular depolarization. It is measured from the onset of the P wave to the beginning of the QRS complex. The normal value is in the range of 0.12–0.20 s and is related to heart rate; the slower the heart rate, the longer the PR interval.

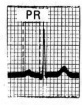

**QRS interval** (Fig 3–5): This is the ventricular depolarization time. It is measured from the onset of the Q wave (or R if no Q is visible) to the termination of the S wave. The upper limit of normal is 0.10 s in frontal plane leads and 0.11 s in precordial leads.

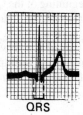

**Figure 3–5.** Normal intervals.

The **ventricular activation time** (VAT) is the time it takes an impulse to traverse the myocardium from endocardial to epicardial surface. It is reflected in clinical electrocardiography by the measurement from the beginning of the Q wave to the peak of the R wave (Fig 3–6). The VAT should not exceed 0.03 s in $V_{1-2}$ and 0.05 s in $V_{5-6}$.

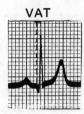

**Figure 3–6.** Ventricular activation time.

**QT interval** (Fig 3–7): This is measured from the onset of the Q wave to the end of the T wave and represents the duration of electrical systole. The QT interval varies with the heart rate and with autonomic nervous system input. The QT interval may be corrected for heart rate ($QT_c$) (Fig 3–8), but this rate correction does not take into consideration autonomic tone, which may not vary directly with the heart rate. The normal $QT_c$ usually does not exceed 0.42 s in men and 0.43 s in women.

On occasion, the end of the T wave is not well seen, or a U wave may be superimposed upon the T wave. Measurement of the QT interval under these circumstances cannot be made with precision. If a portion of the downstroke of the T wave is visible, extrapolation of a line of this slope to the baseline will give a reasonable approximation of the QT interval. The QT interval should be measured in those electrocardiographic leads that display the best-defined T waves.

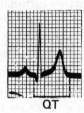

**QU interval** (Fig 3–7): This measures the interval from the beginning of the Q wave to the end of the U wave. It measures total ventricular repolarization time, including that of the Purkinje fibers. When the end of the T wave is not well demarcated because of superimposition of a U wave, the QTU interval may be measured in place of the QT interval.

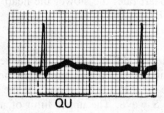

**Figure 3–7.** QRST–U intervals.

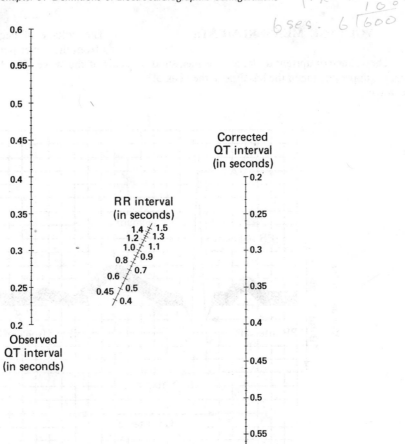

**Figure 3–8.** Nomogram for rate correction of the QT interval. Measure the QT and the RR intervals. Mark these values in the respective columns of the chart. Place a ruler across these 2 points. The point at which the extension of this line crosses the third column is read as the corrected QT interval (QT$_c$). (Reproduced, with permission, from Kissin et al: *Am Heart J* 1948;**35**:990.)

## NORMAL SEGMENTS & JUNCTIONS

**PR segment** (Fig 3–9): That portion of the electrocardiographic tracing from the end of the P wave to the onset of the QRS complex. It is normally isoelectric.

**RST (J) junction:** The point at which the QRS complex ends and the ST segment begins.

**RST segment (usually called the ST segment):** That portion of the tracing from the J point to the onset of the T wave. This segment is usually isoelectric but may vary from −0.5 to +2 mm in precordial leads. It is elevated or depressed in comparison with that portion of the baseline between the end of the T wave and the beginning of the P wave (TP segment) or when related to the PR segment.

**TP segment:** That portion of the tracing between the end of the T wave and the beginning of the next P wave. At normal heart rates, it is usually isoelectric.

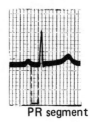

PR segment

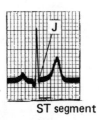

ST segment

**Figure 3–9.** PR and ST segments.

## VOLTAGE MEASUREMENTS

The voltage of upright deflections is measured from the upper portion of the baseline to the peak of the wave.

The voltage of negative deflections is measured from the lower portion of the baseline to the nadir of the wave (Fig 3–10).

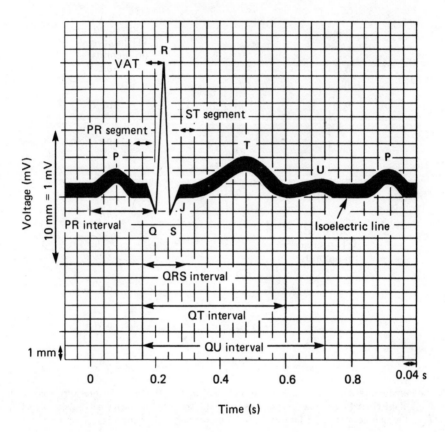

**Figure 3–10.** Diagram of electrocardiographic complexes, intervals, and segments.

# The Cardiac Vector | 4

The term "cardiac vector" designates all of the electromotive forces of the cardiac cycle. A vector has magnitude, direction, and polarity. At any given instant during depolarization and repolarization, electrical potentials are propagating in many directions in space. Over 90% of these potentials are canceled out by opposing forces, and only the net force is recorded. The **instantaneous vector** represents the net electrical force at a given instant. The **mean vector** of a given portion of the depolarization-repolarization sequence (eg, the QRS complex) represents the mean magnitude, direction, and polarity for that time period (eg, the mean QRS vector). The mathematical symbol of a vector is an arrow pointing in the direction of the net potential (positive or negative); the length of the arrow indicates the magnitude of the electrical force. A vector can be drawn for atrial depolarization (P vector), ventricular depolarization (QRS vector), and ventricular repolarization (ST and T vectors).

## FRONTAL PLANE VECTORS

The result of the electrical potentials of the entire cardiac cycle as reflected in the frontal plane of the body is the **frontal plane vector.** By combin-

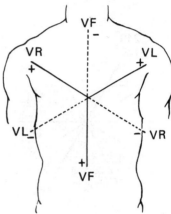

**Figure 4–2.** Frontal plane unipolar leads.

ing the frontal plane bipolar leads I, II, and III (Fig 4–1) with the frontal plane unipolar leads VR, VL, and VF (Fig 4–2), a hexaxial reference system can be drawn that illustrates all 6 leads of the frontal plane (Fig 4–3).

By convention, the positive pole of lead I is designated as 0 degrees and the negative pole as ±180 degrees; the positive pole of VF as +90 degrees and the negative pole as +270 or −90

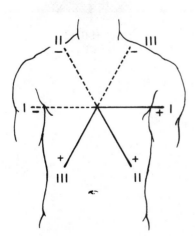

**Figure 4–1.** Frontal plane bipolar leads.

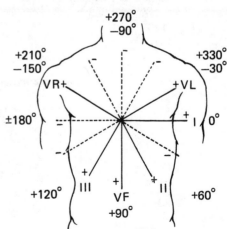

**Figure 4–3.** Frontal plane leads.

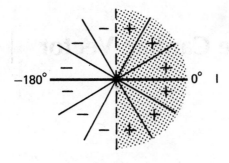

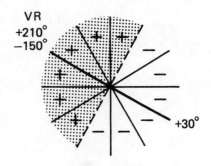

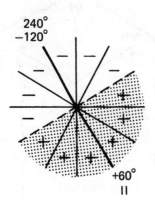

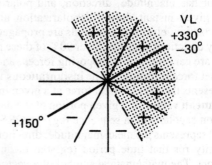

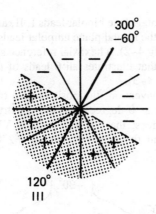

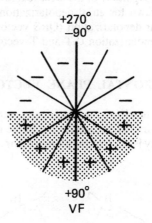

**Figure 4–4.** Polarity of frontal plane lead axis.

degrees; the positive pole of lead II as +60 degrees; the positive pole of lead III as +120 degrees; the positive pole of VR as +210 or −150 degrees; and the positive pole of VL as +330 or −30 degrees.

## Polarity of Individual Frontal Plane Lead Axes

If a perpendicular is drawn through the center of a given lead axis, any electrical force (vector) oriented in the positive half of the electrical field will record an upright deflection in that lead; any force oriented in the negative half of the electrical field will record a downward deflection (Fig 4–4).

## Direction of Mean Frontal Plane Axis

The mean QRS vector in the frontal plane can be approximated from standard leads by use of the hexaxial reference system (Fig 4–3). This is only an approximation, however, since it is determined by measurement of magnitude (voltage) alone, whereas the true mean QRS vector must be determined from both magnitude and time. The net magnitudes and direction of the QRS complexes as in any 2 of the 3 standard leads are plotted along the

axes of the 2 standard leads. Perpendicular lines are drawn at these locations. A line drawn from the center of the reference system to the intersection of the perpendiculars represents the approximate mean QRS vector. Its angle is the frontal plane axis.

Another means of approximating the mean frontal plane QRS axis is as follows: If any one lead of the 6 frontal plane leads has a net QRS magnitude of zero, the mean QRS vector will be perpendicular to that lead axis. Inspection of another lead (I or aVF) will tell in which half of this perpendicular the mean vector is located (Figs 4–5 and 4–6). If no frontal plane lead has a net QRS magnitude of zero, the mean vector can be interpolated and estimated by inspection of several frontal plane leads.

By the same methods, the mean frontal plane axis of the P and the T waves can be determined, as can the angle between the QRS complex and the T wave.

## Axis Deviation

The angle of the mean frontal QRS vector determines its frontal plane axis. The normal QRS axis lies between 0 and +110 degrees; left (supe-

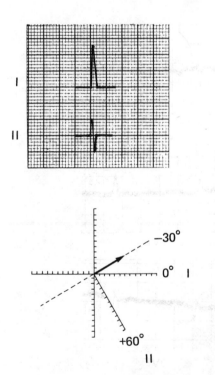

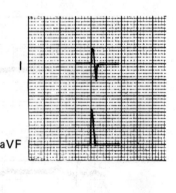

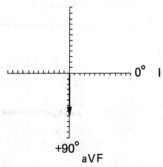

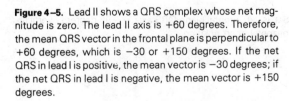

**Figure 4–5.** Lead II shows a QRS complex whose net magnitude is zero. The lead II axis is +60 degrees. Therefore, the mean QRS vector in the frontal plane is perpendicular to +60 degrees, which is −30 or +150 degrees. If the net QRS in lead I is positive, the mean vector is −30 degrees; if the net QRS in lead I is negative, the mean vector is +150 degrees.

**Figure 4–6.** Lead I shows a QRS complex whose net magnitude is zero. The lead I axis is 0 degrees. Therefore, the mean QRS vector in the frontal plane is perpendicular to 0 degrees, which is +90 or −90 degrees. If the net QRS in lead aVF is positive, the mean vector is +90 degrees. If the net QRS in lead aVF is negative, the mean vector is −90 degrees.

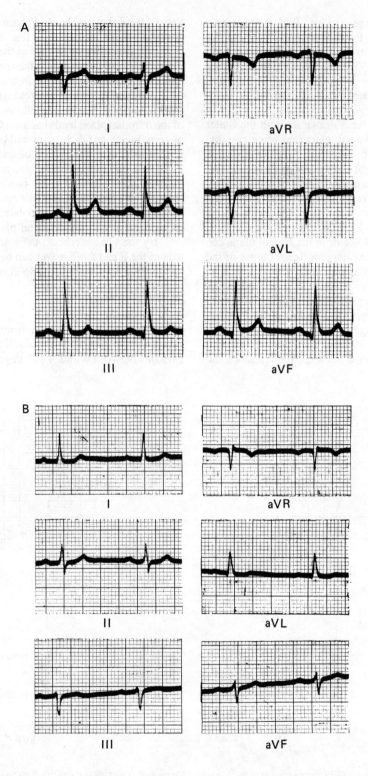

**Figure 4–7.** Examples of normal variations in frontal plane QRS axis. *A:* Frontal plane QRS axis = +96 degrees; vertical heart position. *B:* Frontal plane QRS axis = −10 degrees; horizontal heart position.

rior) axis deviation between −30 and −90 degrees and right axis deviation between +110 and ±180 degrees are abnormal. Within the range of normal, left (superior) axis deviation (0 to −30 degrees) represents a normal horizontal heart position in unipolar terminology, and right axis deviation (+75 to +110 degrees) represents a normal vertical heart position (Fig 4–7). Although the term left axis is traditional, a more accurate term would be **superior axis.**

## HORIZONTAL PLANE VECTORS

The unipolar precordial leads represent approximations of the electrical potentials (vectors) in the horizontal plane (Fig 4–8).

As described for the frontal plane, a perpendicular can be drawn through the zero point of any unipolar precordial lead axis. Any electrical force oriented in the positive half of the electrical field will record a positive (upright) deflection in that lead; any force oriented in the negative half of the electrical field will record a negative (downward) deflection in that lead (Fig 4–9).

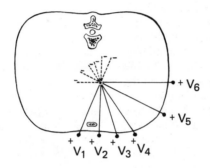

**Figure 4–8.** Lead axes in the horizontal plane.

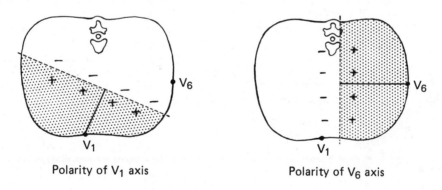

Polarity of V₁ axis

Polarity of V₆ axis

**Figure 4–9.** Polarity of V₁ and V₆ axes.

# Normal Electrocardiographic Complexes

## THE CONDUCTION SYSTEM OF THE HEART

Cardiac muscle has the property of automatic impulse formation and rhythmic contraction. Impulses are formed in specialized tissue that forms the atrioventricular (AV) conduction system. The conduction system consists of the sinoatrial (SA) node (which itself consists of P cells that form the impulse, transitional cells that transmit the impulse through the node, and collagen fibers), interatrial conduction "pathways" (or tracts), the AV node, the bundle of His, the right and left bundle branches, the fascicles of the left bundle branch (anterosuperior, inferoposterior, and septal), and the distal Purkinje system (Fig 5–1).

The rhythm of the heart normally originates in the SA node. The SA node is about 5 × 20 mm and is located at the endocardial surface of the right atrium at the junction of the right atrial appendage

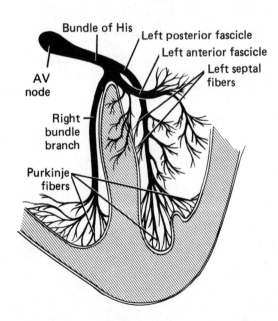

**Figure 5–1.** Illustration of the AV node–His-Purkinje conduction system.

and the superior vena cava. The impulse formed in the SA node is transmitted to atrial muscle via specialized cells, or "pathways" (although they are not clearly anatomically defined as such). The **anterior interatrial pathway** leaves the SA node anteriorly and curves around the superior vena cava and anterior wall of the right atrium, where it divides into 2 bundles: one goes to the left atrium and the other traverses the interatrial septum to the anterosuperior margin of the AV node. The **middle interatrial pathway** leaves the posterior margin of the SA node, curves behind the superior vena cava, and courses along the posterior portion of the interatrial septum to enter the superior margin of the AV node. The **posterior interatrial pathway** leaves the posterior margin of the SA node and courses along the crista terminalis and eustachian ridge to enter the posterior margin of the AV node. Fibers from all 3 pathways converge before entering the AV node; some bypass the AV node to enter the His-Purkinje system distal to the node.

The AV node measures about 2 × 5 mm and is located on the endocardial surface of the right side of the interatrial septum just inferior to the os of the coronary sinus (Fig 5–1). The bundle of His is in direct continuity with the lower portion of the AV node. It is about 20 mm long and is located on the endocardial surface of the right side of the interatrial septum. The bundle of His is divided by collagen septa into longitudinal tracts, which continue into the bundle branches; thus, the bundle branches actually originate in the bundle of His.

The right bundle branch arises from the bundle of His and traverses the endocardial surface of the right side of the interventricular septum (Fig 5–1). It divides into Purkinje fibers quite close to the myocardium. The left bundle branch arises from the bundle of His and divides into 3 radiations, or fascicles. The more proximal is the inferoposterior fascicle, which spreads as a broad band of fibers over the posterior and inferior endocardial surface of the left ventricle. Just distal to the origin of the inferoposterior fascicle is the origin of the anterosuperior fascicle, which spreads as a narrower radiation of fibers over the anterior and superior endocardial surface of the left ventricle. Septal fibers, which do not constitute a well-defined fascicle, spread over the left side of the interventricular septum; there is considerable individual variability in the configuration of the septal fibers.

After traversing the bundle branches, the cardiac impulse enters the peripheral Purkinje system, which covers the endocardial surfaces of both ventricles. It spreads from endocardium to epicardium through the ventricular myocardium.

## ATRIAL COMPLEXES

The P wave represents atrial depolarization. The normal P wave in standard, extremity, and precordial leads does not exceed 0.11 s in duration or 2.5 mm in height. Since the spread of excitation from the SA to the AV nodes is in a leftward and superior-inferior direction, the P wave is normally upright in leads I, II, aVF, and $V_{3-6}$ and normally inverted in aVR (and frequently in $V_1$ and sometimes in $V_2$). It may be upright or inverted in lead III or aVL, depending upon the mean frontal plane P wave axis (Fig 5–2).

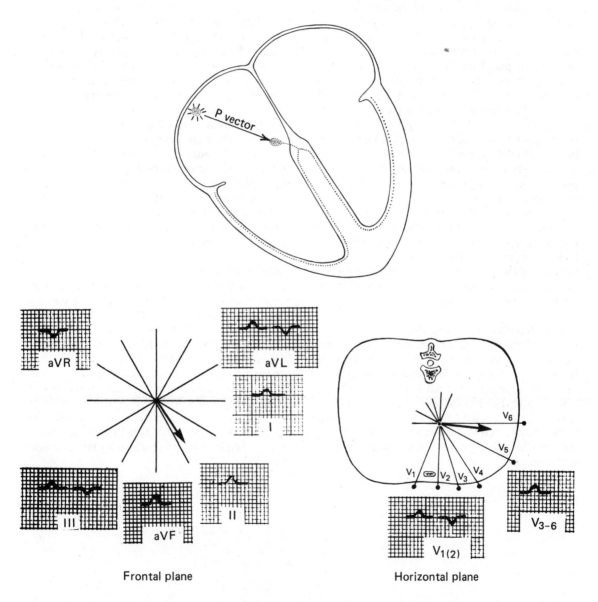

**Frontal plane**            **Horizontal plane**

**Figure 5–2.** Direction of the normal frontal and horizontal plane P wave vectors with the resulting P wave in the 12-lead ECG. The normal P wave vector in the frontal plane is between 0 and +90 degrees. A P wave vector between 0 and +30 degrees will produce an inverted P wave in lead III. A P wave vector past +60 degrees will produce an inverted P wave in lead aVL. The degree of anterior orientation in the horizontal plane will determine whether the P wave is upright or inverted in lead $V_1$.

Atrial repolarization is represented by a wave following the P wave, termed the $T_a$ wave. It is usually best recorded in leads II, III, and aVF when the P waves in these leads are prominent. The $T_a$ wave as recorded in the inferior leads is a broad (up to 0.40 s), negative wave that can occasionally deform the ST segment. Most often, however, the $T_a$ wave is inapparent in the ECG.

## VENTRICULAR COMPLEXES

The QRS complex represents ventricular activation. Initial depolarization of the ventricles occurs across the mid portion of the interventricular septum from left to right. The impulse then passes down the right and left bundle branches and fascicles into the peripheral Purkinje system, initiating activation in the ventricles. The myocardium is depolarized from the endocardial to the epicardial surface. Since the muscle mass of the left ventricle is much greater than that of the right ventricle, there will be greater electrical potential spreading through the left ventricle compared to the right ventricle. The last portions of ventricular muscle to be depolarized are the posterobasal portion of the left ventricle, the area of the pulmonary conus, and the uppermost portion of the interventricular septum.

Repolarization follows depolarization and is a complex event that remains poorly understood. It is known that the ventricular cavities are negative during repolarization; the epicardial surface of the left ventricle is positive and that of the right ventricle is either positive or negative.

### Septal Depolarization (Fig 5–3)

Activation of the septum from left to right results in a vector oriented to the right and anteriorly. The vector is of short duration (usually less than 0.01 s) and is of small magnitude (0.1–0.2 mV). It contributes to the normal small q waves in leads I and $V_{5-6}$ and the r wave in $V_{1-2}$. The septal vector may be oriented inferiorly or superiorly; in the latter instance, a small q wave in aVF will be inscribed.

### Early Activation of the Anteroseptal Region of the Myocardium (Fig 5–4)

The resulting vector is oriented in a direction similar to that of septal depolarization. It is also of short duration and small magnitude and further contributes to the q wave in leads I and $V_{5-6}$ and r wave in $V_{1-2}$.

### Major Activation of the Right & Left Ventricles (Fig 5–5)

Since the left ventricle is dominant in the normal adult, the mean forces will be oriented to the left, posteriorly, and usually inferiorly. This vector will produce a dominant R wave in lead I and $V_{5-6}$. The actual morphology of the QRS complexes in leads II, III, aVL, and aVF will depend upon the frontal plane QRS axis. Lead $V_1$ will record a small r wave with a deeper S wave (R:S ratio less than 1). As one progresses from $V_1$ to $V_6$ the R waves become larger and the S waves smaller.

### Late Activation of the Posterobasal Portion of the Left Ventricle, Pulmonary Conus, & Uppermost Portion of the Interventricular Septum (Fig 5–6)

The mean vector is often oriented to the right, producing small s waves in leads I and $V_{5-6}$. In 5% of normal adults it is directed anteriorly, producing small r' waves in $V_{1-2}$.

### Ventricular Repolarization (Fig 5–7)

In the normal adult, ventricular repolarization results in an isoelectric ST segment and a mean T wave vector oriented to the left, inferiorly (between 0 and +90 degrees in the frontal plane), and slightly anteriorly. This produces upright T waves in leads, I, II, and aVF and inverted T waves in aVR. The polarity of the T wave in leads III and aVL will depend upon the mean frontal plane T wave axis. If it is between 0 and +30 degrees, it will normally be inverted in lead III; if it is between +60 and +90 degrees, it will be inverted in lead aVL. The T wave may be upright or inverted in lead $V_1$ but is upright in leads $V_{2-6}$.

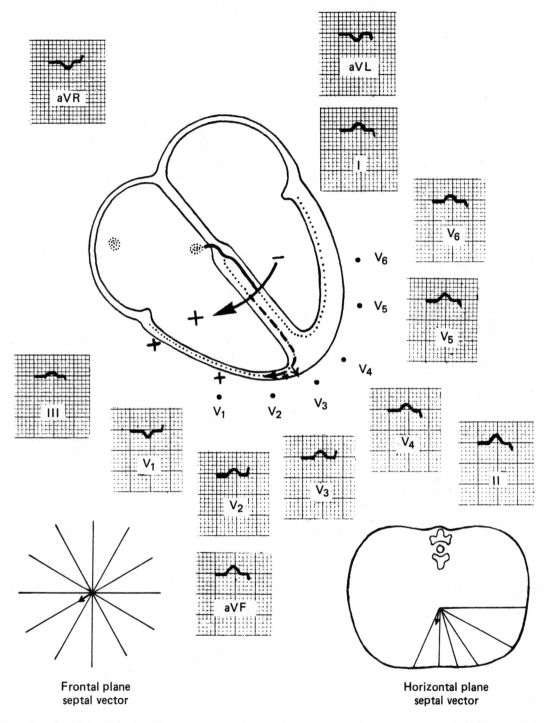

Frontal plane
septal vector

Horizontal plane
septal vector

**Figure 5–3.** Septal depolarization. The vector of septal depolarization is directed rightward and anteriorly. This results in a positive deflection (r wave) in lead $V_1$ and a negative deflection (q wave) in left ventricular epicardial leads (such as $V_5$).

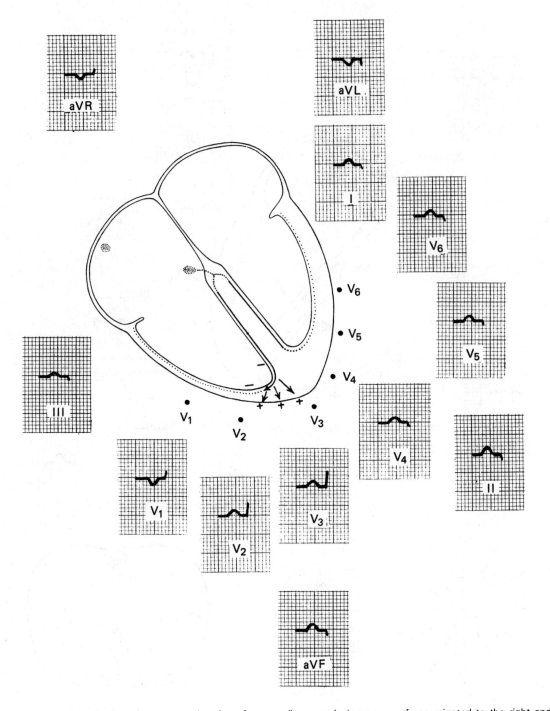

**Figure 5—4.** Early activation of anteroseptal region of myocardium, producing a mean force oriented to the right and anteriorly.

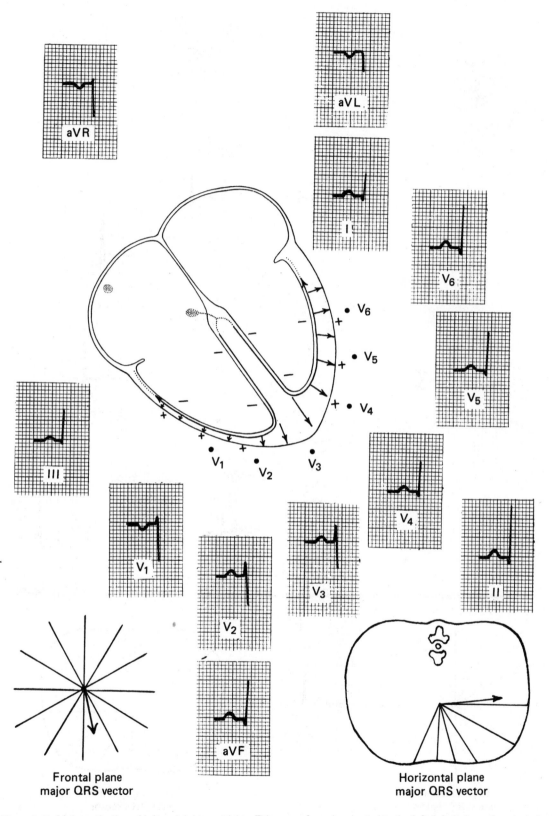

**Figure 5–5.** Major activation of left and right ventricles. This mean force is oriented to the left, inferiorly, and posteriorly.

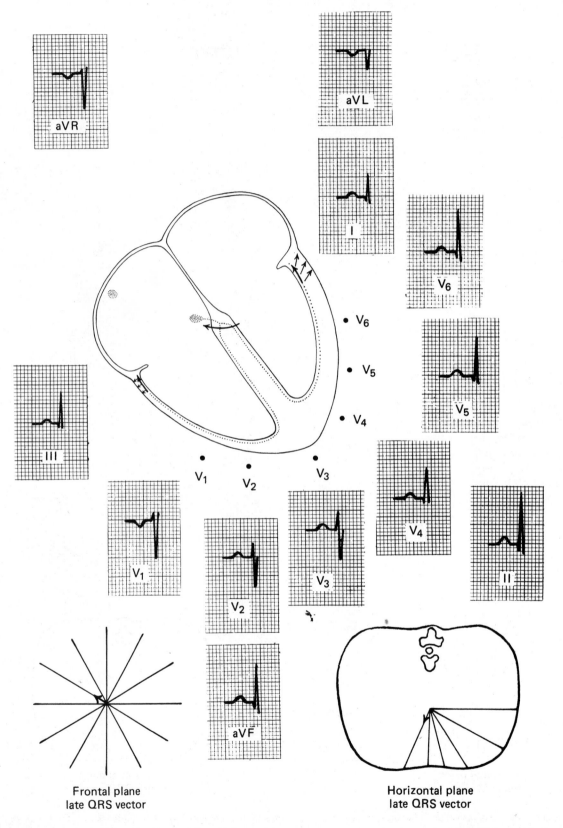

Frontal plane
late QRS vector

Horizontal plane
late QRS vector

**Figure 5–6.** Activation of posterobasal portion of left ventricle, pulmonary conus, and uppermost portion of interventricular septum. The mean force is oriented rightward, superiorly, and anteriorly.

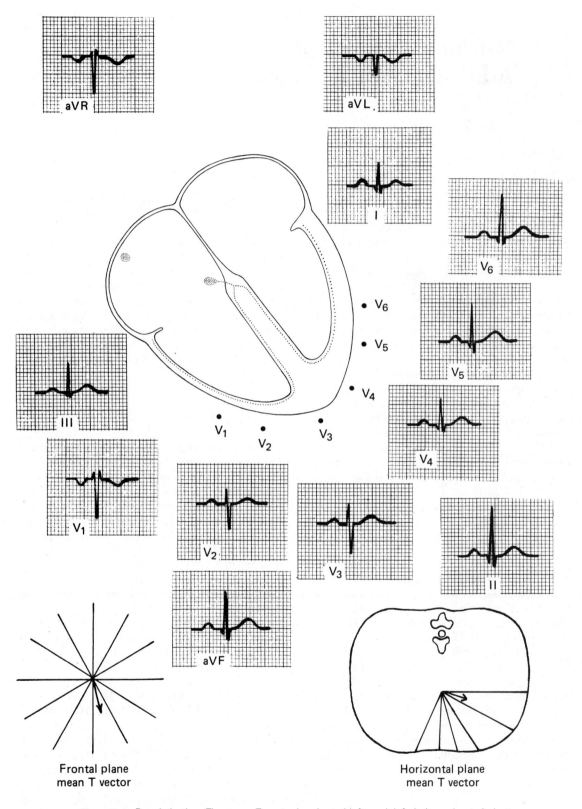

**Figure 5–7.** Repolarization. The mean T vector is oriented leftward, inferiorly, and anteriorly.

# 6 | Normal Variants of the Adult Electrocardiogram

"Normal" electrocardiographic measurements are determined from studies of large groups of clinically normal individuals. Using the 100th percentile range for each measurement, wide overlap between normal and abnormal measurements would render electrocardiographic interpretation practically worthless. Thus, arbitrary limits of "normality" are in the 95th to 98th percentile range. Therefore, for any given electrocardiographic measurement, 2–5% of normal persons will fall outside the normal range and be considered to have abnormal ECGs.

Recognized sources of variability in the ECG include age, sex, body weight, chest configuration, position of the heart within the thoracic cage, race, food intake, exercise, smoking, and position of the precordial leads. Ideally, the patient should be at rest for 15 minutes prior to recording an ECG, should not have had a recent meal, and should not have smoked for 30 minutes. Reproducibility of precordial lead placement should be ensured by proper attention to correct positioning and, when indicated, by marking the precordial positions on the chest wall with ink.

## ST SEGMENT ELEVATION

The ST segment may be elevated up to 2 mm in the precordial leads in normal persons. Occasionally, up to 4 mm of ST segment elevation can occur in left precordial leads (Fig 6–1). The elevated ST segment occurring in a normal individual has an upward concave configuration, and the T wave is usually upright. During exercise, the elevated ST segments usually become isoelectric (Fig 6–1).

ST segment elevation in normal persons is considered to represent early repolarization of a portion of the ventricular myocardium, occurring before depolarization is completed in other areas of the myocardium.

## ST SEGMENT ELEVATION & T WAVE INVERSION

As a further variant of the above pattern, late T wave inversion can be seen in those leads that record the ST segment elevation (Fig 6–2). This combination of ST–T wave abnormalities may simulate myocardial disease and indicates the mandatory requirement for clinical correlation. For unknown reasons, ST elevation with T wave inversion is more common in blacks. With exercise and the concomitant sinus tachycardia, these changes are normalized.

## HYPERVENTILATION

In normal subjects who have episodic anxiety and hyperventilation, several abnormalities of the ECG have been described, including PR interval prolongation, sinus tachycardia, and ST segment depression with or without T wave inversion. These findings are most often recorded in leads II, III, aVF, and left precordial leads. The electrocardiographic abnormalities may simulate myocardial ischemia but have been documented to occur in individuals with no heart disease and normal coronary arteriograms. The abnormalities have been considered to be due, at least in part, to imbalance of autonomic nervous system input. Drugs such as atropine, propranolol, and potassium can result in normalization of the ECG (Fig 6–3).

## EFFECT OF FOOD INTAKE ON THE ELECTROCARDIOGRAM

Following a heavy meal, especially one of high carbohydrate content, ST depression or T wave inversion (or both) may occur. This represents a physiologic (not a pathologic) phenomenon and is due in part to an intracellular shift of potassium in association with intracellular glucose metabolism. Such electrocardiographic changes may simulate a variety of pathologic states (Fig 6–4).

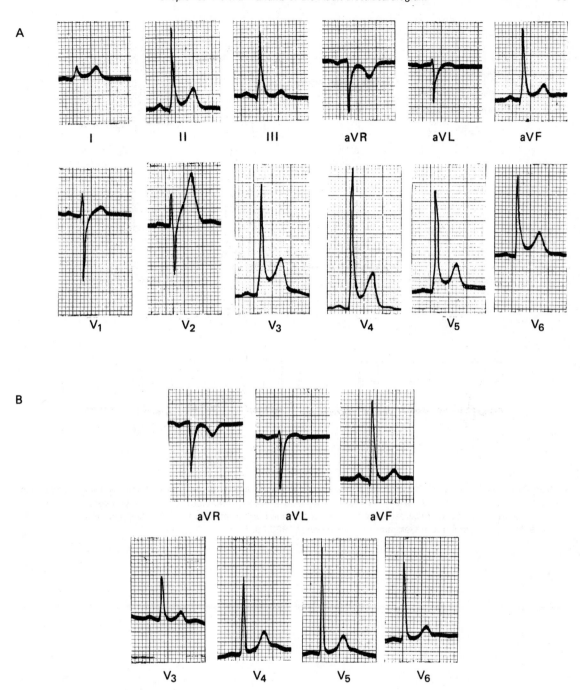

**Figure 6–1.** ST segment elevation in a normal person, occurring as a normal variant. *A:* The resting ECG shows marked ST segment elevation in $V_{3-5}$, reaching 4 mm in $V_{3-4}$. *B:* After exercise, the ST segment approaches the isoelectric baseline.

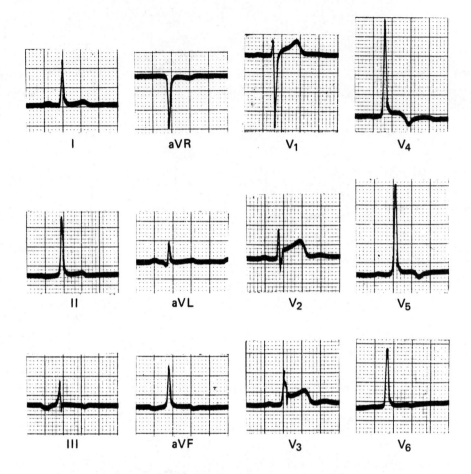

**Figure 6–2.** ST segment elevation with T wave inversion as a normal variant, recorded in a 23-year-old healthy black man. These ST–T wave abnormalities were not modified by mild exercise, beta-blocking drugs, hyperventilation, or vagal blocking agents. Whereas submaximal exercise may not result in normalization of the ST–T findings, maximal effort can temporarily abolish them. (From Goldman MJ: *Am Heart J* 1960;**59**:71.)

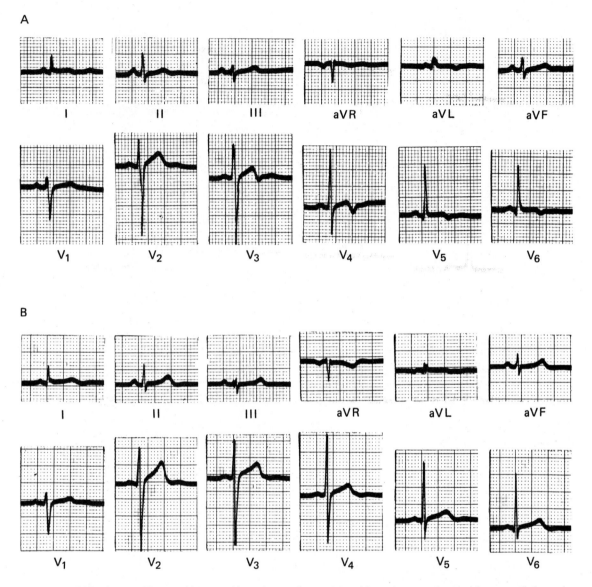

**Figure 6–3.** ECGs from a 26-year-old man without heart disease but with anxiety reaction and hyperventilation. *A:* Abnormal "resting" ECG shows inverted T waves in $V_{4-6}$. *B:* After intravenous atropine, the ECG is normal.

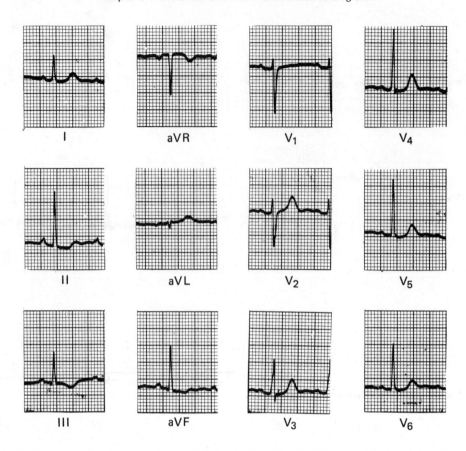

**Figure 6–4.** Nondiagnostic ST and T wave abnormalities in a healthy 30-year-old woman who had eaten a heavy meal 60 minutes earlier. A repeat ECG taken 3 hours postprandially was entirely normal.

## EFFECT OF DEEP RESPIRATION ON THE ELECTROCARDIOGRAM

While not strictly speaking a "normal variant" of the ECG, substantial changes in individual electrocardiographic leads during deep respiration develop in some patients (Fig 6–5). These changes

occur because the position of the heart within the chest cage becomes more vertical with deep inspiration and horizontal with deep expiration. Variations in right and left ventricular stroke volume during respiration may also play a role in these electrocardiographic changes.

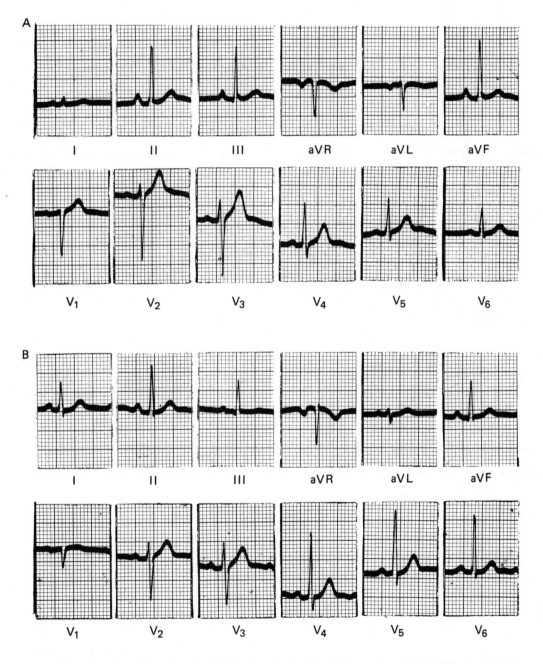

**Figure 6–5.** Effect of deep respiration on the ECG. *A:* Deep inspiration. The mean frontal plane QRS axis is +85 degrees, and the heart position is vertical. *B:* Deep expiration. The heart position is now more horizontal, and the mean frontal plane QRS axis is +65 degrees. There is greater QRS voltage in lead I, less negative voltage in aVL, a decrease in voltage in aVF, and an increase in voltage in $V_{4-6}$ during expiration.

## TEST TRACINGS

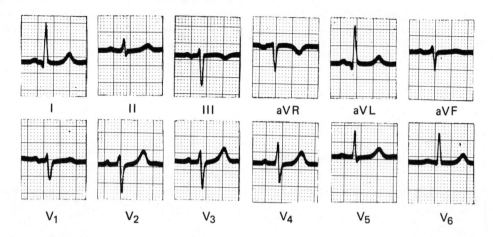

**Figure 6–T1.** Normal ECG. PR interval = 0.14 s; QRS duration = 0.08 s; mean frontal plane QRS axis = −20 degrees. Horizontal heart position.

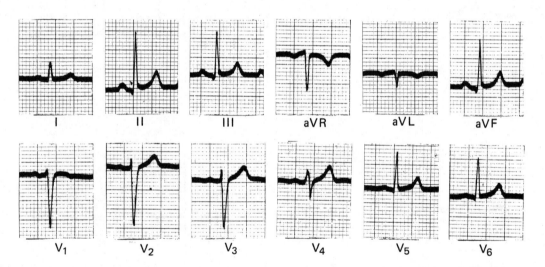

**Figure 6–T2.** Normal ECG. PR interval = 0.14 s; QRS duration = 0.08 s; mean frontal plane QRS axis = +70 degrees. Vertical heart position.

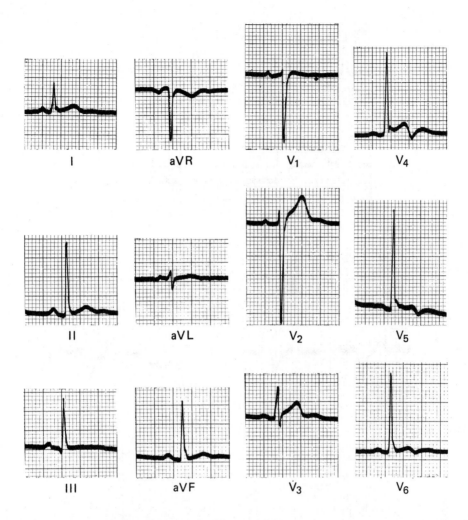

**Figure 6–T3.** Normal variant ECG in a healthy 24-year-old black man. The frontal plane leads are within normal limits. ST segment elevation is present in $V_{2-5}$ and late T wave inversion in leads $V_{4-6}$. There is a prominent precordial voltage. No clinical evidence of left ventricular hypertrophy was present.

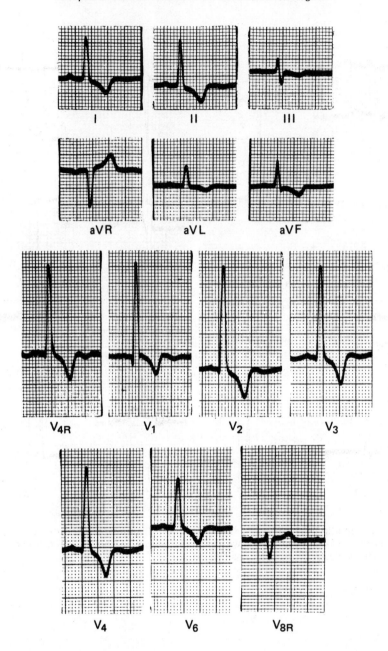

**Figure 6–T4.** Anatomic rotation of the heart on its horizontal axis due to congenital dextroversion. The mean frontal plane QRS axis is +30 degrees. ST segment depression and T wave inversion are present in leads I, II, aVL, and aVF. Very tall R waves with ST depression and T wave inversion are seen in leads $V_{4R}$ through $V_5$, suggesting the possibility of right ventricular hypertrophy. However, the presence of dextroversion, in which the left ventricle is the anterior ventricle, invalidates these criteria.

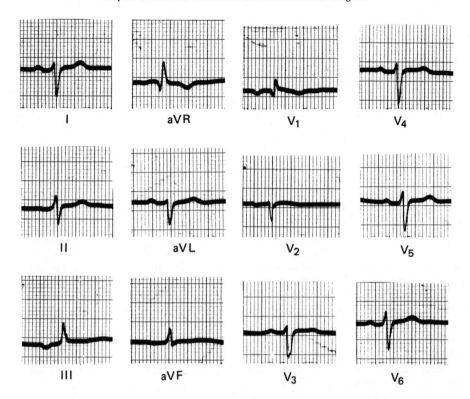

**Figure 6–T5.** Anatomic rotation of the heart on its horizontal axis due to congenital absence of the left pericardium, an anomaly that allows the heart to be displaced to the left, resulting in the major QRS forces being oriented rightward and posteriorly. The mean frontal plane QRS axis is +15 degrees, a QR complex is present in $V_1$, and deep S waves persist through $V_6$. The criteria for right ventricular hypertrophy are invalid in the presence of anatomic rotation of the heart.

# 7 | Hypertrophy

## ATRIAL HYPERTROPHY

The normal P wave does not exceed 0.12 s in width and 2.5 mm in height. An increase in these values suggests the presence of atrial abnormality—which could be hypertrophy, enlargement, conduction delay within the atria, or a combination of these. Inasmuch as the ECG does not distinguish among these conditions, the term **atrial abnormality** is preferred to **atrial hypertrophy.** Where additional electrocardiographic evidence for atrial hypertrophy exists—as, for example, when the pattern of ventricular hypertrophy is present—the diagnosis of atrial hypertrophy is more certain. Similarly, when electrocardiographic evidence of myocardial infarction or intraventricular conduction system disease is present, left atrial enlargement and interatrial conduction delay are more likely diagnoses, respectively, than is atrial hypertrophy. Thus, electrocardiographic evidence of a single entity causing the abnormalities in P wave configuration should be sought.

### Left Atrial Abnormality
The criteria for left atrial abnormality are (1) a broad (≥ 0.12 s), notched P wave usually best seen in leads I and II, with (2) a wide (1 mm × 0.04 s) terminal negative deflection in lead $V_1$. The early portion of the P wave represents right atrial depolarization and the latter portion left atrial depolarization (Fig 7–1). Hypertrophy or enlargement of the left atrium results in an accentuation of the left atrial portion of the P wave, producing a broad, notched wave in the standard leads. Since the left atrium lies posterior to the right atrium, depolarization of a hypertrophied or enlarged left atrium will produce the prominent negative component of the P wave in the right precordial leads (Fig 7–2).

### Right Atrial Abnormality
The criteria for right atrial abnormality are (1) tall, peaked P waves in leads II, III, and aVF (≥ 2.5 mm in height in lead II) (Fig 7–3) and (2) prominent peaked, diphasic, or markedly inverted P waves in lead $V_1$. The P wave duration is normal, and the mean P wave vector in the frontal plane is between +75 and +90 degrees.

### "Pseudo-P-Pulmonale"
This term denotes a prominent P wave in leads

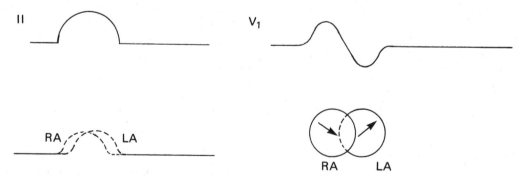

**Figure 7–1.** Diagram of atrial depolarization in relation to the P wave inscribed in leads II and $V_1$ of the surface ECG. The initial portion of the P wave results from right atrial depolarization, and the latter portion of the P wave results from left atrial depolarization. Enlargement or hypertrophy of either chamber will result in accentuation of that portion of the P wave to which it contributes most. In lead II, left atrial abnormality will result in a broad, notched P wave, and right atrial abnormality will result in a tall P wave. In precordial lead $V_1$, left atrial abnormality will result in a prominent terminal negative component of the P wave associated with a posteriorly directed depolarization, and right atrial abnormality will cause a tall, peaked initial portion of the P wave.

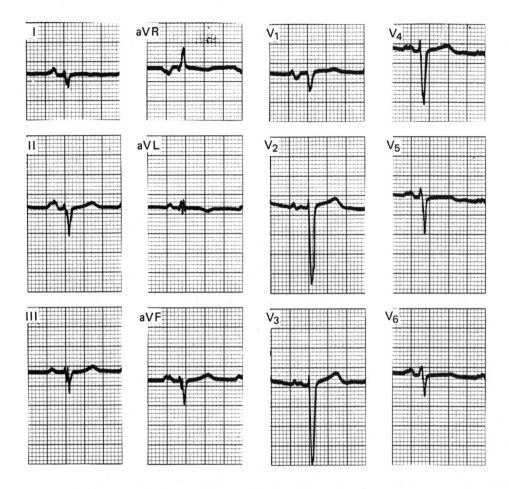

**Figure 7–2.** Left atrial abnormality characterized by broad, notched P waves best seen in leads II, aVF, and $V_{2-5}$ and by a prominent (1 mm × 0.04 s) terminal negative deflection in lead $V_1$. The frontal plane QRS axis is −150 degrees, and S waves are present in I, II, and III, suggesting right ventricular hypertrophy. In view of the possibility of right ventricular hypertrophy, a diagnosis of left atrial hypertrophy could be made. The patient had mitral stenosis.

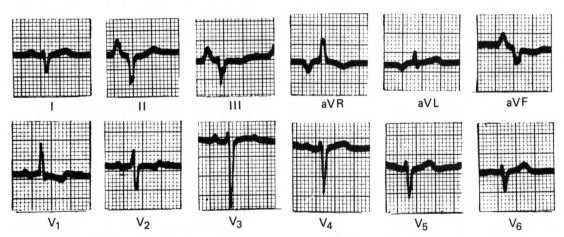

**Figure 7–3.** Right atrial and right ventricular hypertrophy. The P waves are abnormally tall in leads II, III, and aVF, indicating right atrial abnormality. The frontal plane QRS axis is oriented rightward (deep S in I) and superiorly (QS complexes in II, III, and aVF); the axis is −110 degrees. A tall R wave is present in $V_1$. The rightward axis and tall R wave in $V_1$ indicate right ventricular hypertrophy. In the presence of right ventricular hypertrophy, QS complexes need not indicate myocardial infarction.

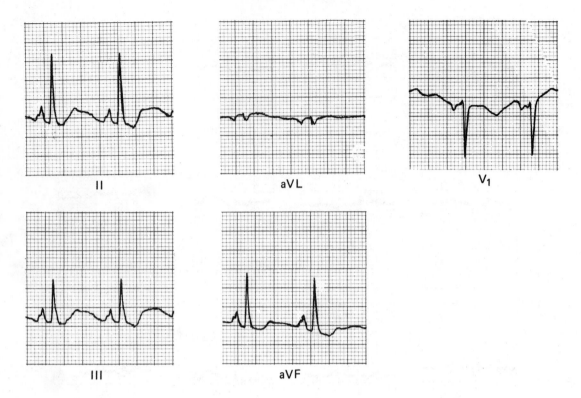

**Figure 7–4.** "Pseudo-P-pulmonale." The P waves appear markedly tall in leads II, III, and aVF. However, the initial (right atrial) portion of the P wave is normal; thus, the prominence is due to a left atrial abnormality, which is confirmed by the deep, wide negative P wave component in lead $V_1$.

II, III, and aVF that is due to left rather than right atrial abnormality. The genesis of this wave is accentuation of that portion of the P wave which reflects left atrial depolarization, ie, the latter portion of the P wave (Fig 7–1). The initial portion of the P wave, reflecting right atrial depolarization, is normal. Depolarization of a severely diseased left atrium results in a tall terminal portion of the P wave. Involvement of the left atrium in production of the pseudo-P-pulmonale pattern is confirmed by identifying the deep, wide negative component of the P wave in lead $V_1$ (Fig 7–4).

## $T_a$ Waves

$T_a$ waves are waves of atrial repolarization (Fig 7–5). While a normal feature of some ECGs, this wave is accentuated in atrial hypertrophy or enlargement and in conditions that cause atrial injury, such as pericarditis or atrial infarction. A prominent $T_a$ wave can mimic a q wave of myocardial infarction or pericarditis by causing depression of the PR segment (Fig 7–5). If the $T_a$ wave is of long duration, it can also mimic ST segment scooping or depression.

## VENTRICULAR HYPERTROPHY

Ventricular hypertrophy develops as a result of pressure or volume load imposed upon the ventricles. A correlation exists between the thickness of ventricular muscle and the magnitude of its depolarization wave (the R wave), although the underlying reasons are far from clear. In addition to—and in part because of—the increased muscle mass in ventricular hypertrophy, there is delay in conduction of impulses through the hypertrophied chamber and often an alteration in the depolarization and repolarization pathways. Thus, the electrocardiographic features of ventricular hypertrophy are (1)

**Figure 7–5.** Prominent atrial repolarization ($T_a$) waves, producing pronounced PR segment depression.

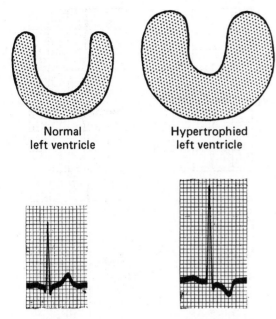

**Figure 7–6.** Diagram of a normal and a hypertrophied left ventricle and the associated QRS complexes recorded from overlying electrocardiographic leads. Compared to the normal QRS complex, the QRS complex recorded over the hypertrophied ventricle has greater height, prolonged intrinsicoid deflection (ventricular activation time), ST segment depression, and asymmetrical T wave inversion.

**Table 7–1.** Summary of electrocardiographic criteria for left ventricular hypertrophy.

**I. Precordial Leads:**
  A. R waves in $V_5$ or $V_6$ over 27 mm. S in $V_1$ + R in $V_5$ or $V_6$ over 35 mm (over 35 years of age).
  B. VAT over 0.05 s in $V_{5-6}$.
  C. QRS interval may be prolonged over 0.1 s.
  D. ST segment depression and T wave inversion in $V_{5-6}$.

**II. Frontal Plane Leads:**
  A. Horizontal Heart: R wave of 11 mm or more in aVL (except when frontal plane axis is superior to −30 degrees); VAT, QRS interval, and ST−T changes as described for precordial leads. $R_1$ + $S_3$ over 26 mm; pattern in I similar to aVL.
  B. Vertical Heart: R wave of over 20 mm in aVF; VAT, QRS interval, and ST−T changes as described for precordial leads. Unless confirmed by precordial leads, this pattern in aVF is not diagnostic of left ventricular hypertrophy (since right ventricular hypertrophy can give a similar pattern in aVF).

**Minimal Criteria**

R in aVL greater than 11 mm; or R in $V_{5-6}$ greater than 27 mm; or S in $V_1$ + R in $V_{5-6}$ greater than 35 mm.

an increase in the height of the R wave, (2) prolongation of the QRS duration, (3) lengthening of the activation time (intrinsicoid deflection) over the hypertrophied ventricle, (4) ST segment depression, and (5) T wave abnormalities consisting typically of asymmetric inversion, which may be shallow or deep (Fig 7–6). Those leads reflecting the electrical potentials recorded from sites opposing the hypertrophied ventricle will show (1) a deep S wave or QS complex, (2) an elevated ST segment, and (3) an upright T wave.

### Left Ventricular Hypertrophy (Table 7–1)

Left ventricular hypertrophy may result from a variety of conditions (Table 7–2). The electrocardiographic abnormalities may precede the radiologic changes and thus may be the first clue to the diagnosis.

The mean frontal plane QRS axis is often deviated to the left, to between 0 and −30 degrees. If the leftward axis deviation exceeds −30 degrees, concomitant left anterior fascicular block may be present (see Chapter 8).

A left ventricular epicardial complex is recorded in extremity lead aVL. A tall R wave with a depressed ST segment and an inverted T wave will

therefore be seen in this lead (Fig 7–7). An R wave equal to or exceeding 11 mm in lead aVL is highly specific for the diagnosis of left ventricular hypertrophy (although it is an insensitive marker, occurring in only about 25% of cases), provided that the mean frontal plane QRS axis is not pathologically deviated to the left. In the presence of abnormal left axis deviation (superior to −30 degrees), left ventricular hypertrophy is suggested (but not proved) when the height of the R wave exceeds 16 mm (Fig 7–8).

Tall R waves with depressed ST segments and inverted T waves will also be seen in precordial leads $V_{4-6}$. The QRS duration may exceed 0.10 s, and the ventricular activation time may be greater then 0.05 s. Deep S waves will be present in anterior

**Table 7–2.** Common causes of left ventricular hypertrophy.

(1) Hypertension
(2) Valvular aortic stenosis
(3) Hypertrophic cardiomyopathy
    Concentric
    Asymmetric
(4) Supravalvular aortic stenosis
(5) Aortic regurgitation
(6) Mitral regurgitation
(7) Coarctation of the aorta
(8) Patent ductus arteriosus
(9) "Athletic heart"

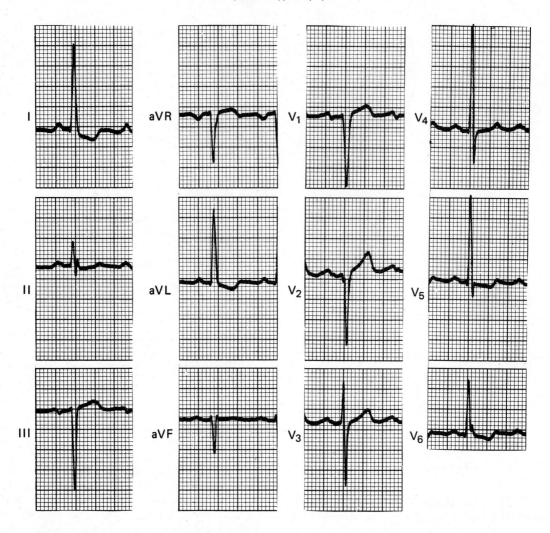

**Figure 7–7.** Left ventricular hypertrophy. The mean frontal plane QRS axis is −15 degrees. The R wave exceeds 15 mm in aVL, and the sum of the S wave in $V_1$ and the R wave in $V_5$ exceeds 35 mm. ST segment depression is present in leads I and aVL, and T wave inversion is present in I, aVL, and $V_{5-6}$. The deep S waves in the right precordial leads reflect the large electrical force generated by the hypertrophied left ventricle. The ST segment elevation in $V_{1-2}$ is consistent with left ventricular hypertrophy.

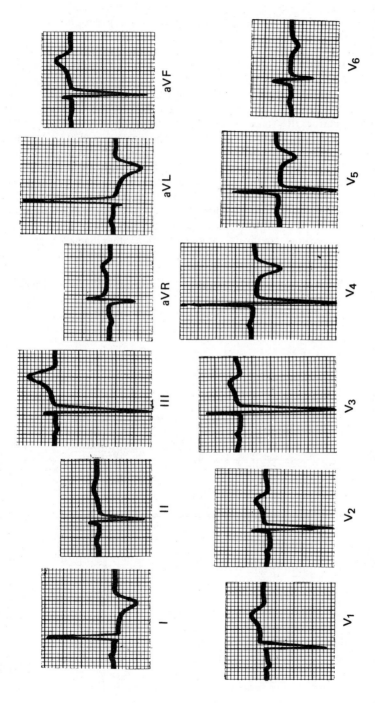

**Figure 7–8.** Left ventricular hypertrophy with left (superior) axis deviation. The mean frontal plane QRS axis is −45 degrees, suggesting the possibility of left anterior fascicular block. The R wave of 24 mm in aVL, however, strongly suggests (but does not prove) the presence of left ventricular hypertrophy. ST segment depression and T wave inversion are present in aVL, and T wave inversion is present in $V_{4-6}$. Precordial lead voltage criteria for left ventricular hypertrophy are not met. This may be due to the superior axis, as a result of which the lead axes of $V_{5-6}$ are far removed from the mean QRS vector. Left ventricular hypertrophy was confirmed at autopsy examination.

precordial leads $V_{1-2}$, since these right precordial leads reflect the greater potential generated by the thick left ventricle. As a general rule, left ventricular hypertrophy is present if the voltage of $SV_1 + RV_5$ or $SV_1 + RV_6$ exceeds 35 mm or if the R wave in $V_5$ or $V_6$ exceeds 27 mm. However, prominent precordial voltage alone (without concomitant ST and T wave abnormalities) is an insufficient criterion for the diagnosis of left ventricular hypertrophy, since large voltages may be recorded in normal young adults and thin-chested individuals.

In patients with marked left ventricular hypertrophy, and especially in those with septal hypertrophy, there can be loss of anterior QRS forces (small or absent r waves in $V_{1-3}$), mimicking anterior wall myocardial infarction. Less commonly, abnormal Q or QS waves can be recorded in the inferior leads (II, III, and aVF) or lateral leads (I and $V_6$), simulating inferior or lateral wall myocardial infarction.

Some patients with left ventricular hypertrophy have hearts that are oriented vertically in the chest. The mean frontal plane QRS axis in such patients may be normal rather than leftward, and prominent voltage is present in leads II, III, and aVF (Fig 7–9). Precordial lead voltage criteria for left ventricular hypertrophy, along with the associated ST and T wave abnormalities, may be applied in making the correct diagnosis.

## Right Ventricular Hypertrophy (Table 7–3)

Right ventricular hypertrophy may result from several common clinical conditions (Table 7–4). In right ventricular hypertrophy, the mean frontal plane QRS axis may be normal or deviated to the right. Axis deviation to the right of +110 degrees in an adult suggests the presence of right ventricular hypertrophy provided that left posterior fascicular block (see Chapter 8) is not present. In standard leads II and III and in extremity lead aVR, tall R waves are seen; in aVR, this may be a QR, qR, or R complex. The right precordial leads typically show tall R or qR waves with prolonged ventricular activation time. QR or qR waves in aVR or $V_1$ may reflect a delay in activation of the hypertrophied right ventricle (such that early left ventricular depolarization is recorded) and depolarization of a hypertrophied interventricular septum in a superior-inferior direction rather than a left-to-right direction (or both). Although the QRS duration may be slightly prolonged, it does not exceed 0.12 s. ST segment depression and T wave inversion are inscribed in the right precordial leads (Fig 7–10). Since prominent voltage in leads II, III, and aVF

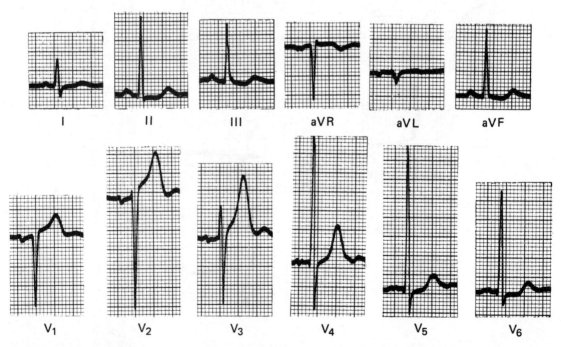

**Figure 7–9.** Left ventricular hypertrophy in a patient with a normal mean frontal plane QRS axis of +75 degrees. There are tall R waves in II, III, and aVF. The sum of $SV_1 + RV_5 = 55$ mm, and ST depression is present in $V_{5-6}$. The P waves are notched in all leads, suggesting left atrial hypertrophy. Prominent precordial voltage associated with a normal or rightward deviation of the mean frontal plane QRS axis should also raise the suspicion of biventricular hypertrophy.

**Table 7—3.** Summary of electrocardiographic criteria for right ventricular hypertrophy.

**I. Precordial Leads:** These are the best leads for diagnosis.
  A. R wave of greater voltage than S wave in $V_1$ or $V_{3R}$.
  B. qR pattern in $V_1$ or $V_{3R}$.
  C. VAT over 0.03 s in $V_1$ or $V_{3R}$.
  D. Persistent S waves in $V_{5-6}$.
  E. ST segment depression and T wave inversion in $V_{1-3}$.

**II. Frontal Plane Leads:**
  A. Right axis deviation (greater than or equal to +110 degrees); depressed ST and inverted T in II and III.
  B. Tall R in aVR; unless accompanied by the criteria in I, this alone is not indicative of right ventricular hypertrophy.
  C. Tall R with depressed ST and inverted T in aVF; unless confirmed by precordial leads, this pattern itself is not diagnostic of right ventricular hypertrophy.

**Minimal Criteria**

Rs or qR complex in $V_1$ or $V_{3R}$ with VAT greater than 0.03 s. Right axis deviation.

**Helpful (But Not Diagnostic) Criteria**

Abnormally tall or notched P waves; ST depression with T wave inversion in $V_{3R}$ and $V_{1-3}$ in the absence of a tall R in these leads; right intraventricular conduction delay.

**Table 7—4.** Common causes of right ventricular hypertrophy.

(1) Chronic obstructive pulmonary disease
(2) Pulmonary hypertension
    Primary
    Pulmonary emboli (acute, massive)
    Pulmonary emboli (chronic, recurrent)
    Mitral stenosis
    Mitral regurgitation
    Chronic left ventricular failure
(3) Tricuspid regurgitation

In the absence of a conduction delay involving the right ventricle, tall R wave voltage in the right precordial leads is helpful in diagnosing right ventricular hypertrophy. A better criterion, however, is the R:S ratio in lead $V_1$: This is normally less than 1.0 in the adult, but as the right ventricle hypertrophies some of the leftward forces normally recorded in the right precordial leads are canceled, resulting in an R:S ratio that approaches or exceeds 1.0. In addition to an abnormal R:S ratio in $V_1$, the R wave decreases in amplitude and the S wave increases in amplitude as the left precordial leads are recorded, reflecting prominent right ventricular forces.

## Electrocardiographic Variations in Right Ventricular Hypertrophy

Not infrequently, the criteria for the diagnosis of right ventricular hypertrophy are not met in patients with clinical evidence of this condition, and the reasons are not entirely understood. Occasionally, a tall, peaked P wave in the inferior leads —

may be seen in patients with left ventricular hypertrophy and a vertically oriented heart, confirmation in the right precordial leads must be sought to diagnose right ventricular hypertrophy with more certainty.

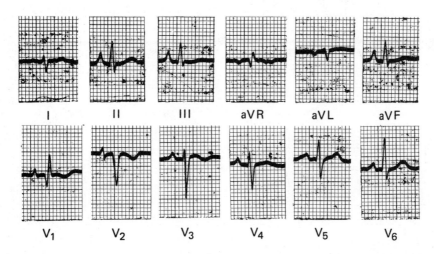

**Figure 7—10.** Right ventricular hypertrophy in a patient with emphysema and right heart failure. The mean frontal plane QRS axis is deviated to the right at +105 degrees. A QR complex is inscribed in aVR and $V_1$. The T waves are inverted in $V_{1-3}$. Right atrial hypertrophy is suggested by the tall, peaked P waves in II, III, aVF, and $V_1$.

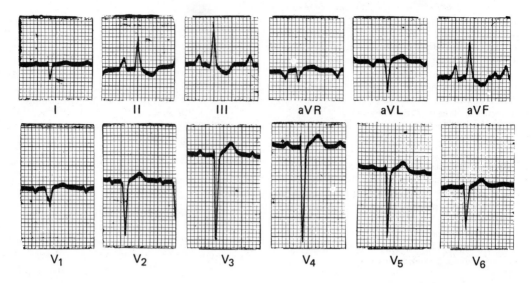

**Figure 7–11.** Probable right ventricular hypertrophy in an older man with pulmonary emphysema. The frontal plane QRS axis is +115 degrees. Tall, peaked P waves are present in II, III, and aVF, suggesting right atrial hypertrophy. QS complexes are present in $V_{1-2}$, and persistent S waves are seen in the left precordial leads. Old anterolateral wall myocardial infarction must be excluded on clinical grounds (see Chapter 10).

which indicates right atrial abnormality (hypertrophy)—may be indirect evidence of right ventricular hypertrophy (which must be inferred) (Fig 7–11).

Although the mean frontal plane QRS axis is deviated to the right in older patients with chronic lung disease and cor pulmonale, it may be directed not anteriorly but posteriorly—resulting in normal, small, or even absent R waves in the right precordial leads (Fig 7–11). In these cases, anterior wall myocardial infarction may be mimicked. The T wave inversion in leads $V_{1-3}$ that may also be seen can further mimic anterior wall ischemia or infarction. As a general rule, when the diagnosis of cor pulmonale due to chronic obstructive lung disease is known, the electrocardiographic diagnosis of myo-

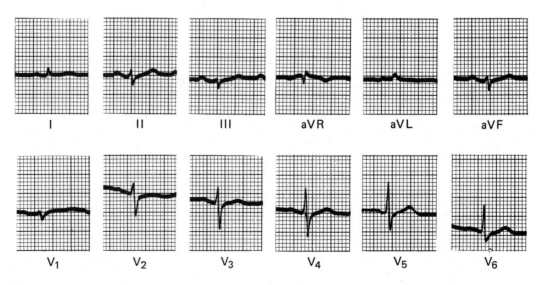

**Figure 7–12.** Possible right ventricular hypertrophy in a patient with pulmonary emphysema. The QRS complexes are of low voltage (none exceeds 5 mm in the standard leads). The mean frontal plane QRS axis is −35 degrees, indicating a leftward and superior direction of depolarization. S waves are seen in $V_{5-6}$ and may be due in part to the superior axis deviation.

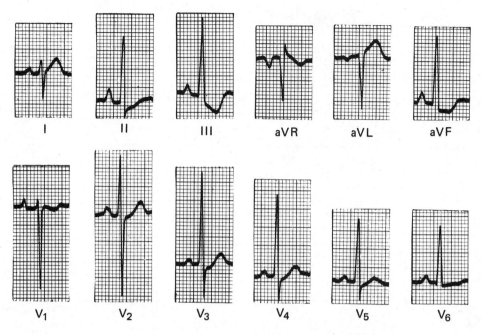

**Figure 7–13.** Combined right and left ventricular hypertrophy. The mean frontal plane QRS axis is +105 degrees. ST segment depression is present in leads II, III, aVF, and $V_6$. $SV_1 + RV_5 = 39$ mm. The combination of right axis deviation and precordial lead voltage criteria for left ventricular hypertrophy is a reliable indicator of biventricular hypertrophy.

cardial infarction should not be made without clinical correlation.

Patients who have emphysema with hyperinflation of the lungs may have ECGs that show diffuse low voltage (due to the hyperinflated lung tissue), where no QRS complex exceeds 5 mm in height; terminal QRS forces in the frontal plane that are directed rightward (S wave in I) and superiorly (S waves in II, III, and aVF); or terminal QRS forces in the frontal plane that are directed leftward (R wave in I) and superiorly (S waves in II, III, and aVF), resulting in superior axis deviation (Fig 7–12). It is important to realize that when the diagnosis of pulmonary emphysema is known, superior deviation of the mean frontal plane QRS axis does not connote disease in the intraventricular conduction system (left anterior fascicular block) but is, rather, a (poorly understood) feature of the lung disease.

## Combined Right & Left Ventricular Hypertrophy

The electrocardiographic diagnosis of ventricular hypertrophy is not perfectly correlated with ventricular weights as determined at autopsy. Whereas a correct electrocardiographic diagnosis of left ventricular hypertrophy can be made 85% of the time using the criteria given above, a false-positive diagnosis is made 10–15% of the time. False-positive diagnoses are more likely if voltage criteria alone (without concomitant ST and T wave abnormalities) are applied in the electrocardiographic interpretation. The correlation of the electrocardiographic diagnosis of right ventricular hypertrophy with autopsy findings is not as good as for left ventricular hypertrophy, ranging from 23 to 100% (the latter in patients with congenital heart disease). Correlation of the electrocardiographic diagnosis of combined ventricular hypertrophy with autopsy results is quite poor, with an accuracy of only 8–26%; thus, this diagnosis cannot be made from the ECG with certainty. The poor correlation is better understood if one recognizes that in biventricular hypertrophy an increase in left ventricular forces counterbalances an increase in right ventricular forces (and vice versa); thus, the mean forces may be those of the left ventricle—or neither ventricle, if left and right ventricular hypertrophy are "balanced."

The most reliable criteria for the electrocardiographic diagnosis of biventricular hypertrophy are the *combination* of right axis deviation (exceeding +90 degrees) in the frontal plane and precordial lead voltage criteria for left ventricular hypertrophy (Fig 7–13).

## TEST TRACINGS

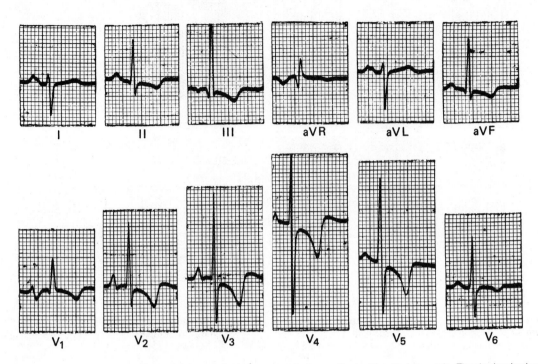

**Figure 7–T1.** Left atrial hypertrophy and right ventricular hypertrophy in a patient with mitral stenosis. The rhythm is sinus, the PR interval = 0.18 s, and the QRS duration = 0.08 s. The mean frontal plane QRS axis is +125 degrees. The P waves are broad and notched in leads I and aVL, and there is a prominent terminal negative deflection in $V_1$, indicating left atrial hypertrophy. The rightward deviation of the frontal plane QRS axis, the qR complex in $V_1$, and the persistent S wave in $V_6$ (with ST depression in $V_{2-5}$) indicate right ventricular hypertrophy.

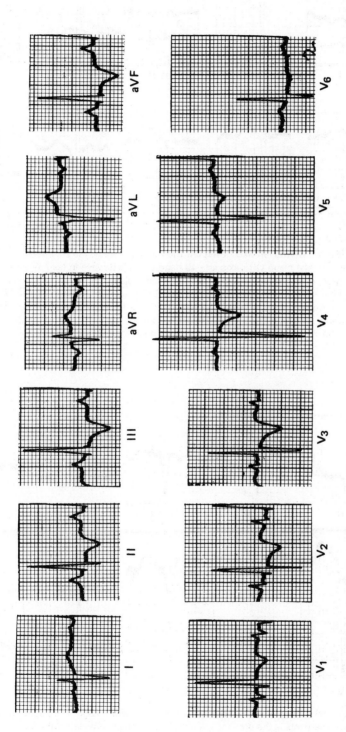

**Figure 7–T2.** Right atrial and right ventricular hypertrophy in a patient with schistosomiasis, pulmonary involvement, and cor pulmonale. The PR interval = 0.16 s, and the QRS duration = 0.09 s. The mean frontal plane QRS axis = +110 degrees. The P waves are tall and of normal duration in II, III, and aVF and sharply diphasic in $V_1$. A qR complex is present in $V_1$. There is ST depression and T wave inversion in II, III, aVF, and $V_{1-5}$.

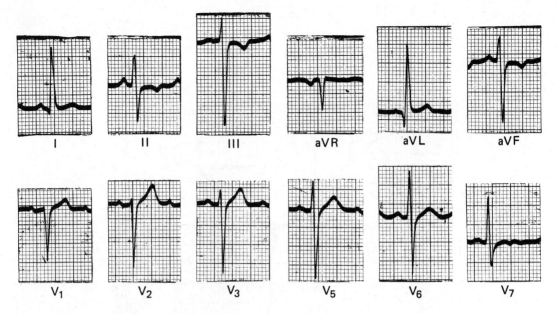

**Figure 7–T3.** Left ventricular hypertrophy with left axis deviation. The rhythm is sinus, the PR interval = 0.14 s, the QRS duration = 0.10 s, and the mean frontal plane QRS axis is −40 degrees. The R wave in lead aVL is 17 mm, which is abnormally tall for this minor degree of leftward deviation of the mean frontal plane QRS axis. The precordial leads show S waves in $V_{5-6}$, which result from the superior (and posterior) mean QRS forces. Whereas left ventricular hypertrophy is often accompanied by left axis deviation, voltage criteria for left ventricular hypertrophy cannot be applied if the axis deviation represents a primary abnormality of the intraventricular conduction system. Without serial ECGs, it is often difficult to tell which process—the ventricular hypertrophy or the axis deviation—came first.

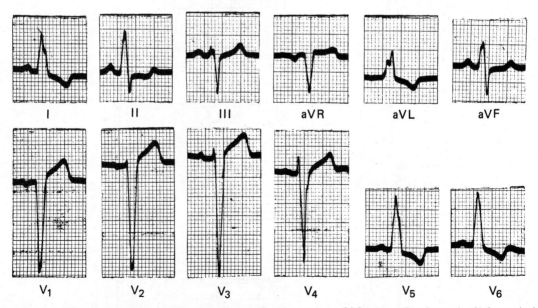

**Figure 7–T4.** Left bundle branch block pattern (see Chapter 8) with prominent QRS voltage. The diagnosis of left ventricular hypertrophy cannot be made with certainty in the presence of a depolarization abnormality of the left ventricular myocardium. The rhythm is sinus, the PR interval = 0.16 s, the QRS duration = 0.12 s, and the mean frontal plane QRS axis is 0 degrees. There are wide, notched R waves in leads I, aVL, and $V_{5-6}$, and the intrinsicoid deflection in lead aVL is 0.10 s. There are secondary ST–T wave abnormalities in left ventricular leads, reflecting the left ventricular depolarization abnormality.

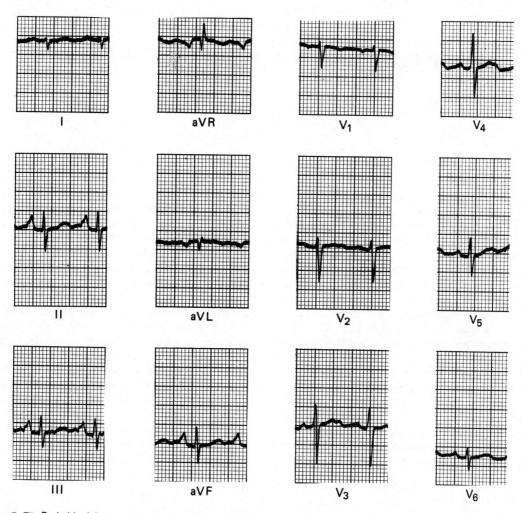

**Figure 7–T5.** Probable right ventricular hypertrophy. The P waves are tall and peaked in II, III, and aVF, consistent with right atrial abnormality (hypertrophy). There are small initial QRS forces directed leftward (r in I) and greater terminal forces directed rightward (S in I); the terminal forces are directed superiorly (S in II, III, and aVF). S waves persist in the left precordial leads, in part because of the superior axis deviation. The patient had emphysema and cor pulmonale.

# 8 | Intraventricular Conduction Delays

An intraventricular conduction delay is the result of impaired impulse conduction through one or more of the divisions of the intraventricular conduction system distal to (or within the lower portion of) the bundle of His (Fig 8–1). The conduction fibers that participate in the depolarization of ventricular tissue are the right bundle branch, the common left bundle branch, and the anterosuperior and inferoposterior radiations (fascicles) of the left bundle branch; there are also septal fibers originating from the left bundle branch, but these do not constitute a true fascicle because of their variability. Thus, the intraventricular conduction system of the heart is a quadrifascicular one (Fig 8–1).

Intraventricular conduction delays are commonly referred to as "blocks" and are classified as "incomplete" or "complete," indicating different degrees of conduction delay. "Incomplete bundle branch block" refers to a conduction delay within a portion of the intraventricular conduction system that does not result in abnormal prolongation of the QRS interval; "complete bundle branch block" refers to a conduction delay that does result in abnormal lengthening of the QRS interval. Neither of these terms is accurate, however. "Block" in a conduction fiber should serve to indicate only that a conduction *delay* is present, not to indicate total inability of an impulse to be transmitted through that fiber. The differential diagnosis of conduction block versus conduction delay cannot be determined by the ECG. Similarly, the terms "incomplete" and "complete" are misleading in that they refer only to lesser and greater degrees of conduction delay rather than to the presence or absence of conduction. Although these terms continue to be used, it must be emphasized that they have no anatomic counterpart and describe conduction *patterns* only.

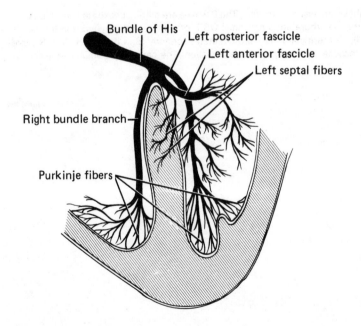

**Figure 8–1.** Diagrammatic illustration of the AV node–His-Purkinje conduction system.

As a result of conduction delay within a fascicle, there is delay of excitation and abnormal spread of excitation through the portion of ventricular muscle served by that fascicle. Therefore, the QRS duration may be prolonged to 0.12 s or longer; the QRS morphology becomes abnormal; the ventricular activation time (the time from onset of the QRS complex to the peak of the R wave) over the involved ventricle becomes prolonged; and the ST segments are depressed and the T waves inverted in leads recording the abnormal depolarization. Lesser degrees of conduction delay produce less prolongation of the QRS duration and ventricular activation time but similar QRS–T morphology.

## RIGHT BUNDLE BRANCH BLOCK PATTERN

The pattern of right bundle branch "block" is a common electrocardiographic finding; although it often occurs in the presence of heart disease of various causes, it is not diagnostic of cardiac disease.

### Mechanism of Impulse Transmission

The spread of excitation from the SA node to the AV node through the main portion of the bundle of His is normal. Activation of the interventricular septum occurs in normal fashion, from left to right.

Left ventricular depolarization occurs in a normal fashion, so the initial 0.04–0.06 s of the QRS complex is normal. Because of the right intraventricular conduction delay (which could be located in the distal portion of the His bundle, the proximal portion of the right bundle branch, or the Purkinje fibers of the right ventricle), right ventricular depolarization is delayed (Fig 8–2).

### Electrocardiographic Pattern (Fig 8–2)

The characteristic feature of right bundle branch block is a late, delayed electrical force of right ventricular depolarization oriented to the right and anteriorly. This late rightward vector produces a wide s wave in leads I and $V_{4-6}$ and a wide R or R' wave in aVR (Fig 8–3). The anterior component of this late force produces the wide R' waves in right precordial leads $V_{3R}$, $V_1$, and $V_2$. This late force may be directed superiorly or inferiorly. If superior, it produces a wide s in aVF; if inferior, it produces a wide R' in aVF. The ST segment and the T wave are opposite in direction to this late force of ventricular depolarization, resulting in ST depression and T wave inversion in right precordial leads $V_{1-3}$. The QRS interval is 0.12 s or greater (Fig 8–3).

If the right bundle branch block is present but the QRS interval is not prolonged beyond 0.12 s, the bundle branch block pattern is described as "incomplete" and indicates a lesser degree of conduction delay (Fig 8–4).

The pattern of septal and left ventricular depolarization in right intraventricular conduction delay is normal. Thus, right bundle branch block does not itself alter the mean frontal plane QRS axis. The mean frontal plane QRS axis should be determined from the initial 0.04–0.06 s of ventricular activation rather than from the entire QRS complex; thus, the duration of the right-sided conduction delay, as measured from the broad s wave in lead I, should be disregarded when determining the axis.

### Right Bundle Branch Block With Left Ventricular Hypertrophy

As right bundle branch "block" reflects delayed activation of the right ventricle, left ventricular events will be not obscured. Thus, the typical characteristics of left ventricular hypertrophy in leads I, aVL, and $V_{4-6}$ will usually be seen (Fig 8–5).

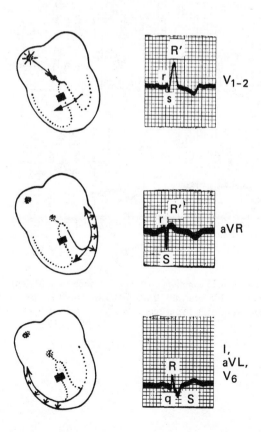

**Figure 8–2.** Right bundle branch block pattern.

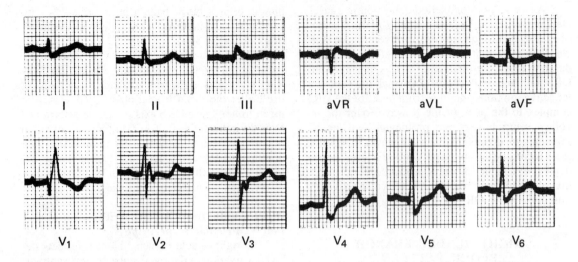

**Figure 8–3.** Right bundle branch block pattern. The mean frontal plane axis of the initial 0.04 s of the QRS complex (measured by subtracting the duration of the wide S wave in lead I) is +60 degrees. The QRS interval is 014 s. The wide s waves in lead I and $V_{4-6}$ and the R' waves in $V_{1-2}$ are typical of right intraventricular conduction delay.

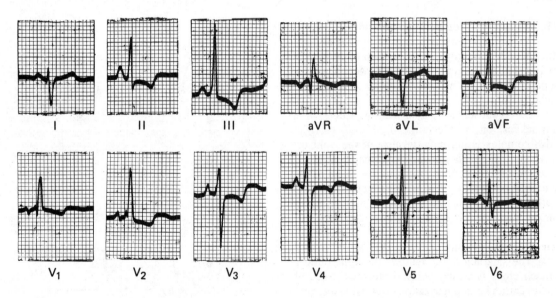

**Figure 8–4.** Incomplete right bundle branch block pattern. The pattern is similar to that of right bundle branch block, except that the QRS interval = 0.08–0.10 s. The right axis deviation (+110 degrees) and the rR' complex in $V_2$ indicate associated right ventricular hypertrophy, and the ST–T wave abnormalities in $V_{2-4}$ are consistent with this diagnosis.

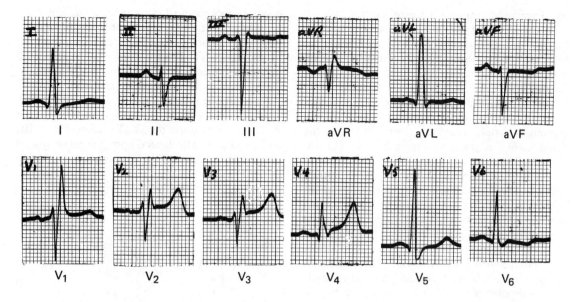

**Figure 8–5.** Right bundle branch block pattern and left ventricular hypertrophy. The precordial leads show the typical pattern of right bundle branch block. The R wave in aVL is 17 mm, indicating left ventricular hypertrophy; the T wave is inverted in V₆, consistent with this diagnosis. The mean frontal plane QRS axis, determined from the first 0.06 s of the QRS complex, is superiorly directed at −50 degrees, consistent with the left ventricular hypertrophy but also possibly reflecting a delay in conduction in the anterior fascicle of the left bundle branch.

## Right Bundle Branch Block With Right Ventricular Hypertrophy

Right ventricular hypertrophy can cause a conduction delay in the right ventricle, much as left ventricular hypertrophy can cause a left-sided conduction delay. However, marked widening of the QRS complex is not usual with hypertrophy alone, and a rightward mean frontal plane QRS axis is not expected from the conduction delay alone. Determination of the initial 0.04- to 0.06-s frontal plane QRS vector is therefore helpful. An abnormal rightward axis (greater than +90 degrees) is consistent with right ventricular hypertrophy (or associated left posterior fascicular conduction delay). In addition, the QRS configuration in lead V₁ is qR or pure R wave in right ventricular hypertrophy (but not in right bundle branch block), in contrast to the rSR′ pattern in right bundle branch block. Finally, the ventricular activation time over the right ventricle (time from onset of QRS complex to peak of the R′ wave) is not markedly delayed in right ventricular hypertrophy, whereas it usually exceeds 0.06 s in right ventricular conduction delay.

## LEFT BUNDLE BRANCH BLOCK PATTERN

The pattern of left bundle branch "block" is more commonly associated with heart disease than is right bundle branch block, but it may also be seen in individuals without evidence of overt heart disease.

## Mechanism of Impulse Transmission

The spread of excitation from the SA node to the AV node and bundle of His occurs in a normal fashion. The impulse is then either not transmitted at all—or is transmitted with delay—in the left bundle branch or fascicles (or both) (Fig 8–1). Since the left septal fibers do not activate the interventricular septum in left bundle branch block, the septum is depolarized from fibers arising in the distal portion of the right bundle branch. This results in a septal vector that is oriented to the left.

The right ventricle is depolarized in normal fashion. The left ventricle is depolarized in an abnormal manner (Fig 8–6). If conduction in the left bundle branch is totally blocked, the left ventricle is depolarized from impulses transmitted from the right bundle branch system across the interventricular septum into the left ventricle. If conduction is delayed in the left bundle branch, the left ventricle will be depolarized by the fibers of the left bundle branch but in a delayed and often abnormal sequence.

## Electrocardiographic Pattern (Fig 8–6)

The abnormal septal depolarization from right to left results in an initial vector oriented to the left. Therefore, the normal q wave is not recorded in leads I and $V_{5-6}$. If q (or Q) waves are recorded in these leads, the possibility of additional disease, such as myocardial infarction, is suggested. In this circumstance, the left ventricular conduction delay is distal to the common left bundle branch (peri-infarction block) (see Chapter 10).

Right ventricular depolarization occurs in a normal fashion, but there is little evidence of this in the conventional ECG, because of the dominance of left ventricular forces. The abnormal left ventricular depolarization results in wide (0.12 s or greater), notched or slurred QRS complexes oriented to the left and posteriorly, typically recorded in leads I and $V_{4-6}$ (Figs 8–6 and 8–7). The polarity of the QRS complexes in leads II, III, and aVF will depend upon the mean frontal plane QRS axis. Since this axis usually lies between 0 and −30 degrees, lead aVL will commonly show the pattern described above.

An abnormal superior axis (above −30 degrees) indicates additional conduction delay in the left anterior fascicle of the left bundle branch. An abnormal rightward axis (greater than +90 degrees) indicates additional conduction delay in the left posterior fascicle of the left bundle branch or associated right ventricular hypertrophy (Fig 8–8). The dominant posterior vector results in small or absent anterior forces in $V_{1-3}$ (producing rS or QS complexes), mimicking anterior wall myocardial infarction. At times, "abnormal" Q waves are recorded in leads III and aVF, but these are not diagnostic of inferior wall myocardial infarction.

As a result of abnormal ventricular depolarization, ventricular repolarization is altered, resulting in *secondary* ST–T wave changes. The ST and T vectors are oriented opposite to the QRS vector. Thus, there is ST depression and asymmetric T wave inversion in leads I and $V_{4-6}$ and elevated ST segments with upright T waves in leads $V_{1-3}$ (Fig 8–7). The direction of the ST–T vectors in leads III, aVF, and aVL will depend upon the mean frontal plane QRS axis and will be opposite to the direction of the QRS vectors.

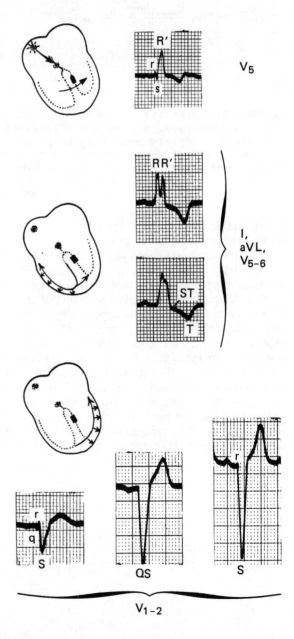

Figure 8–6. Left bundle branch block pattern.

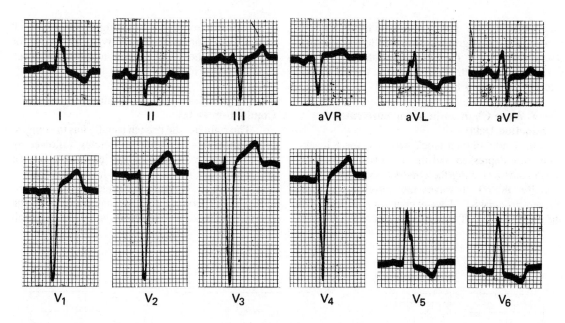

**Figure 8–7.** Left bundle branch block pattern. The mean frontal plane QRS axis is 0 degrees. A wide, notched R wave with depressed ST segment and T wave inversion is seen in leads I, aVL, and V$_{5-6}$. A wide S wave is seen in precordial leads V$_{1-4}$; the ST segments are elevated in V$_{1-3}$ and the T waves are upright. The QRS duration is prolonged to 0.12 s and the ventricular activation time is 0.10 s. Note the absence of Q waves in leads I, aVL, and V$_{5-6}$ caused by right-to-left septal depolarization.

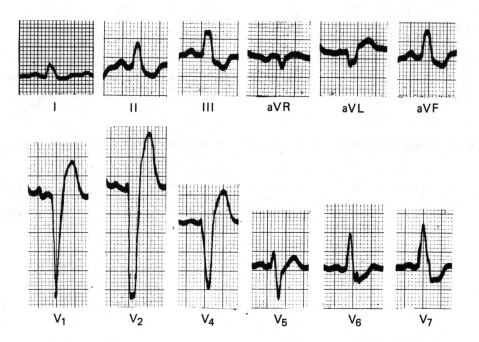

**Figure 8–8.** Left bundle branch block pattern with rightward axis deviation. The mean frontal plane QRS axis is +70 degrees. The QRS morphology is otherwise typical of left intraventricular conduction delay. The rightward axis deviation is presumed to be due to disease in the inferoposterior fascicle of the left bundle branch, resulting in the early forces being oriented in an anterosuperior direction and the late forces in an inferoposterior direction.

"Incomplete" left bundle branch block refers to an electrocardiographic pattern of left-sided conduction delay, but the QRS duration is less than 0.12 s, and the ventricular activation time does not exceed 0.09 s (Fig 8–9).

## ST–T Wave Changes in Intraventricular Conduction Delay

In bundle branch block patterns, the ST segments are depressed and the T waves inverted in those leads reflecting the conduction delay. Occasionally, the ST–T waves are upright, a finding termed *primary* ST–T wave changes, in contrast to the secondary ST–T abnormalities occurring as part

of the conduction delay. Although primary ST–T wave changes are neither sensitive nor specific for myocardial ischemia or infarction, these diagnoses should be considered.

## Rate-Dependent Intraventricular Conduction Delay

The right bundle branch usually has the longest refractory period of all of the fascicles, followed by the left anterior fascicle of the left bundle branch and finally by the left posterior fascicle of the left bundle branch. Premature supraventricular impulses may therefore find various portions of the conduction system refractory when they reach

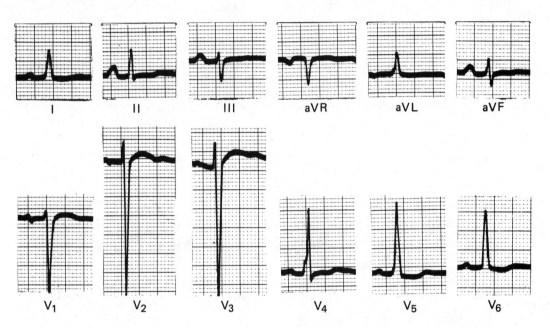

**Figure 8–9.** "Incomplete" left bundle branch block pattern. The QRS duration is 0.10 s. Septal q waves are absent in leads I and $V_{5-6}$. The R wave is slurred in leads I, aVL, and $V_{5-6}$ and notched in $V_4$. ST segment straightening is present in these leads. Precordial voltage criteria for left ventricular hypertrophy are met ($SV_1 + RV_5 = 38$ mm). In tracings such as this one, either the ventricular hypertrophy or the conduction delay has to be assumed to be primary. If ventricular hypertrophy is known to be primary, the conduction delay is presumed to be due to the impulse having to travel through increased ventricular muscle thickness. If, however, the conduction delay is primary, voltage criteria for left ventricular hypertrophy cannot be applied.

them, producing a **rate-dependent conduction delay.** An increase in the atrial rate may also produce this form of intraventricular aberration (Figs 8–10 and 8–11). Rate-dependent bundle branch "block" is a function of the refractory period of conduction tissue, and its occurrence does not imply the presence of heart disease. Following the return of normal intraventricular conduction after a period of bundle branch "block," the T waves of the normally conducted complexes may appear abnormal; the precise mechanism of such T wave abnormalities is not clear, but their occurrence is not predictive of organic heart disease. (Similar T wave abnormalities can follow the appearance of spontaneous QRS rhythm in patients whose sequence of ventricular depolarization has been rendered abnormal by a cardiac pacemaker.)

## Differential Diagnosis of Left Bundle Branch Block & Left Ventricular Hypertrophy

The pattern of left bundle branch block may be seen in the same clinical conditions as those of left ventricular hypertrophy. The major differential point between the 2 electrocardiographic patterns is the absence of a septal q wave in leads that record septal activity in the right-left axis (such as leads I and $V_{5-6}$). The presence of a q wave in these leads is evidence against the diagnosis of left bundle branch block, or it indicates associated infarction. In view of the abnormality of ventricular depolarization, voltage criteria for left ventricular hypertrophy are not valid in the presence of definite left bundle branch "block"; however, extremely prominent voltage might suggest the presence of left ventricular hypertrophy.

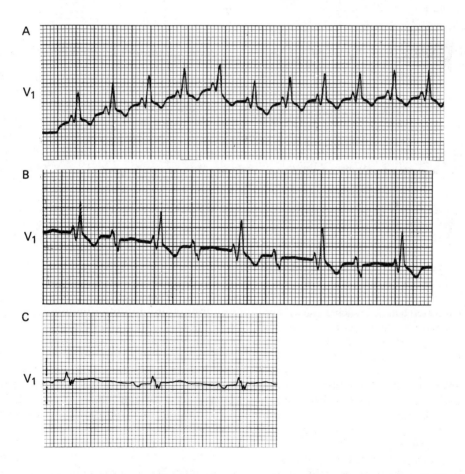

**Figure 8–10.** Rate-dependent right intraventricular conduction delay. *A:* During paroxysmal reciprocating supraventricular tachycardia (see Chapter 11) at a rate of 160/min, the QRS morphology shows a right bundle branch block pattern. (No P waves are visible.) *B:* Several minutes later, the tachycardia rate has slowed to 135/min. QRS complexes having a right bundle branch block pattern alternate at regular intervals with QRS complexes having an RS configuration. *C:* Sinus rhythm, restored several minutes later. The QRS morphology of the sinus-conducted impulses has an RS configuration and is identical to the alternate QRS complexes in (B). Thus, in (B), normal sinus-conducted QRS complexes are alternating with right bundle branch block complexes, indicating 2:1 block in the right bundle branch; in (A), conduction in the right bundle branch did not occur or was delayed.

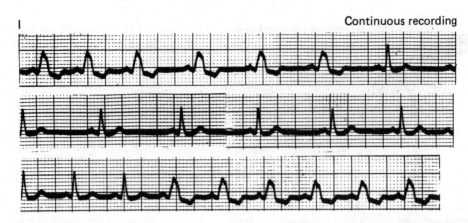

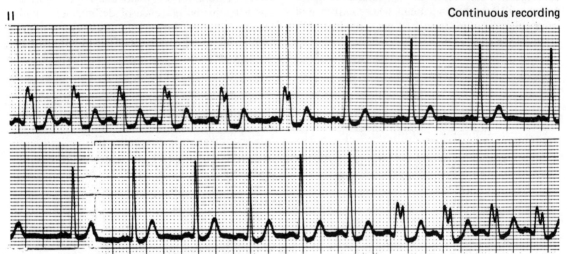

**Figure 8–11.** Rate-dependent left intraventricular conduction delay. At a critical sinus cycle length the left bundle branch is refractory, and the pattern of intraventricular conduction is that of left bundle branch block. Note the disappearance of the septal q wave in lead I (present in the normally conducted complexes) when the left bundle branch block pattern is present.

## FASCICULAR CONDUCTION DELAY

The common left bundle branch divides into its fascicles: the anterior (anterosuperior) fascicle and the inferior (inferoposterior) fascicle (Fig 8–1). The septal fibers are not sufficiently organized to be termed a fascicle. The anterosuperior fascicle radiates out over the anterior and superior surfaces of the left ventricle, and the inferoposterior fascicle radiates out over the inferior and posterior surfaces of the left ventricle. Peripherally, the fibers from both fascicles intertwine.

Normally, impulse transmission proceeds simultaneously down both fascicles, resulting in a normally directed QRS vector in the frontal plane. However, if conduction delay is present in one of the fascicles, the spread of activation proceeds down the normal fascicle first, thus altering the direction of the mean QRS vector in the frontal plane. Since fascicular conduction is so rapid (10–20 ms), the conduction delay is not associated

with measurable prolongation of the QRS complex in the conventional ECG.

Fascicular "blocks" are associated with the inscription of q waves (see below) that, although they might mimic those of myocardial infarction, are not sufficiently wide nor deep to indicate infarction. Should the pattern of preexistent q wave infarction be present, however, and fascicular conduction delay develop, the q waves of infarction may disappear, to be superseded by the depolarization sequence of remaining noninfarcted myocardium.

### Conduction Delay in the Left Anterior Fascicle

Left anterior fascicular conduction delay or "block" results in an abnormal spread of activation through the left ventricular myocardium (Fig 8–12). Ventricular activation initially occurs via the inferoposterior fascicle of the left bundle branch, resulting in a vector oriented inferiorly (r wave in

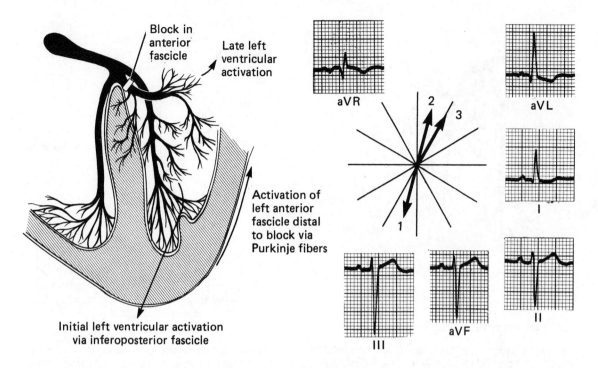

**Figure 8–12.** Left anterior fascicular conduction delay. The initial QRS (arrow 1) is oriented to the right (q in I) and inferiorly (r in II, III, and aVF). The terminal QRS (arrow 2) is oriented to the left (R in I) and superiorly (S in II, III, and aVF). The mean QRS frontal plane vector = −60 degrees (arrow 3).

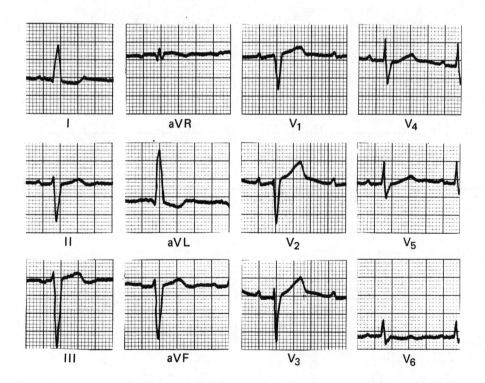

**Figure 8–13.** Left anterior fascicular "block." The mean QRS axis is −50 degrees. The QRS interval is 0.10 s. The R wave voltage in aVL is 14 mm. In the presence of left anterior fascicular "block," this voltage in aVL is not diagnostic of left ventricular hypertrophy. There is ST segment depression in I, aVL, and $V_6$. The small q waves in $V_{1-3}$ are the result of early QRS forces directed inferiorly, rightward, and posteriorly. The s waves in $V_{5-6}$ are the result of the superiorly directed late QRS forces.

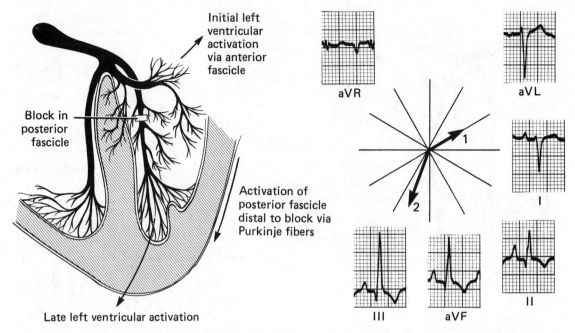

**Figure 8–14.** Left posterior fascicular "block." The initial QRS (arrow 1) is oriented to the left (r in I) and superiorly (q in II, III, and aVF). The terminal QRS (arrow 2) is oriented rightward (S in I) and inferiorly (R in II, III, and aVF), resulting in a mean frontal plane QRS axis of +110 degrees.

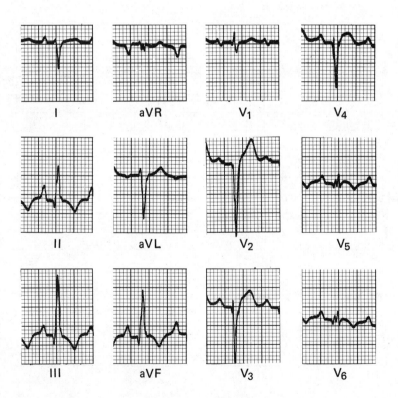

**Figure 8–15.** Left posterior fascicular "block." The mean frontal plane QRS axis is +110 degrees. The QRS interval = 0.1 s. The P waves are tall in II and aVF. The above are consistent with right atrial and right ventricular hypertrophy; however, cardiac catheterization revealed normal right heart pressures. These findings emphasize the necessity for excluding right ventricular hypertrophy before an electrocardiographic diagnosis of left posterior fascicular block is made. The precordial leads are indicative of anterior wall myocardial infarction (see Chapter 10).

leads II, III, and aVF) and rightward (q wave in lead I and, occasionally, small q waves in $V_{2-3}$). Later activation of the ventricle occurs via the fibers of the anterior fascicle, through interconnecting Purkinje fibers distal to the site of conduction delay, resulting in a late vector oriented to the left (R wave in lead I) and superiorly (S waves in leads II, III, and aVF). The mean frontal plane QRS axis is superior to $-30$ degrees (Fig 8–13), although any acute leftward axis shift may indicate some degree of conduction delay in the anterior fascicle. Since Purkinje conduction time is so rapid, the 10–20 ms conduction delay caused by fascicular "blocks" does not produce a measurable increase in the QRS interval. Because the mean QRS vector is directed leftward and superiorly in left anterior fascicular block, voltage criteria for left ventricular hypertrophy using lead aVL cannot be applied. Whether or not precordial lead voltage can be used to diagnose left ventricular hypertrophy has not been definitely established.

## Conduction Delay in the Left Posterior Fascicle

Left posterior fascicular conduction delay or "block" results in abnormal activation of the left ventricle (Fig 8–14). Left ventricular depolarization initially spreads through the anterior fascicle, resulting in a vector oriented to the left (r wave in lead I) and superiorly (q wave in leads II, III, and aVF). Later ventricular activation occurs via fibers from the posterior fascicle, through interconnecting Purkinje fibers distal to the site of conduction delay; this results in a vector oriented to the right (S wave in lead I), inferiorly (R wave in leads II, III, and aVF), and posteriorly (S wave in $V_{1-2}$) (Fig 8–15). The mean frontal plane QRS axis equals or exceeds $+110$ degrees, although any acute rightward shift in axis may indicate some degree of conduction delay in the posterior fascicle.

Left posterior fascicular block occurs only rarely as an isolated finding. The concomitant presence of a right bundle branch block pattern helps to confirm the diagnosis of left posterior fascicular block. Much more common causes of rightward axis deviation are right ventricular hypertrophy and lateral wall myocardial infarction (see Chapter 10).

## Conduction Delay in the Septal Fibers

Normal initial septal depolarization results from impulses transmitted by the septal fibers that arise from the proximal portion of the left bundle branch. The resulting vector is oriented to the right, producing small q waves in leads I and $V_{5-6}$. It might be anticipated that absence of septal q waves would suggest conduction delay in the septal fibers; however, up to 20% of normal individuals do not have septal q waves. This suggests that the interven-

tricular septum may be oriented parallel to the frontal plane of the body. Thus, even though the septum is activated from its left to its right, the projection of this force is anterior but not rightward. Therefore, the diagnosis of "block" in the left septal fibers cannot be made from the ECG.

### Peri-infarction Conduction Delays
See Chapter 10.

## BIFASCICULAR CONDUCTION DELAYS

Bifascicular "block" indicates more diffuse involvement of the intraventricular conduction system by disease. It does not itself predict the development of AV block (see Chapter 12), although the same disease processes that give rise to bifascicular conduction delays can also produce varying degrees of AV block. In acute myocardial infarction, however, the acute development of bifascicular block is of ominous prognostic significance, since it implies extensive necrosis of the septal and ventricular myocardium.

### Right Bundle Branch Block With Left Anterior Fascicular Block

This is one of the most common types of bilateral bundle branch block. It is recognized by the combination of the criteria given above for each type of block: (1) delayed terminal QRS forces oriented to the right and anteriorly, producing wide S waves in I and $V_{5-6}$ and wide R or R′ waves in $V_1$ and $V_2$; plus (2) a mean 0.04- to 0.06-s QRS vector in the frontal plane greater than $-30$ degrees (Fig 8–16).

### Right Bundle Branch Block With Left Posterior Fascicular Block

The electrocardiographic features that permit recognition of this type of bilateral bundle branch block are (1) typical findings of right branch block, and (2) a mean 0.04- to 0.06-s frontal plane QRS axis of $+110$ degrees or greater (Fig 8–17). As in isolated left posterior fascicular block, right ventricular hypertrophy as the cause of the rightward axis must be excluded by clinical evaluation.

## TRIFASCICULAR CONDUCTION DELAYS

Trifascicular conduction delay is suggested by the patterns of bifascicular conduction delay and a prolonged PR interval (Fig 8–18). However, the PR interval includes interatrial conduction, AV nodal

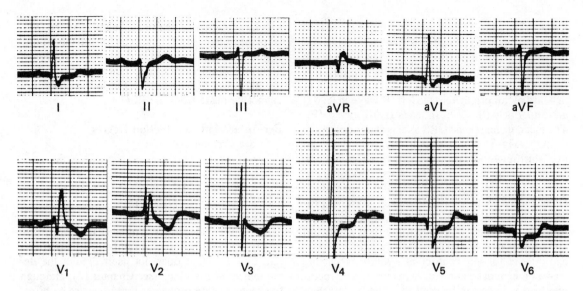

**Figure 8–16.** Bifascicular conduction delays involving the right bundle branch (terminal portion of the QRS oriented to the right and anteriorly, with wide S waves in leads I and $V_{5-6}$ and wide R' waves in $V_{1-2}$) and the left anterior fascicle of the left bundle branch (mean frontal plane QRS axis of −60 degrees). Since right bundle branch block is a terminal conduction delay, the mean forces of left ventricular activation are not obscured by its presence.

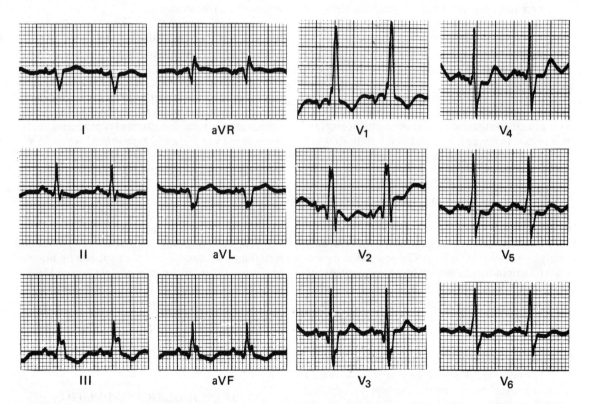

**Figure 8–17.** Bifascicular conduction delays involving the right bundle branch (delayed terminal portion of the QRS, with late orientation to the right and anteriorly, wide S waves in leads I and $V_{5-6}$ and wide, notched R waves in $V_{1-2}$) and the posterior fascicle of the left bundle branch (mean frontal plane QRS axis +120 degrees). The q waves in $V_{1-3}$ indicate anterior wall myocardial infarction—old, as indicated by the upright T waves. Both right ventricular hypertrophy and lateral wall myocardial infarction as causes of the right axis deviation must be excluded on clinical grounds.

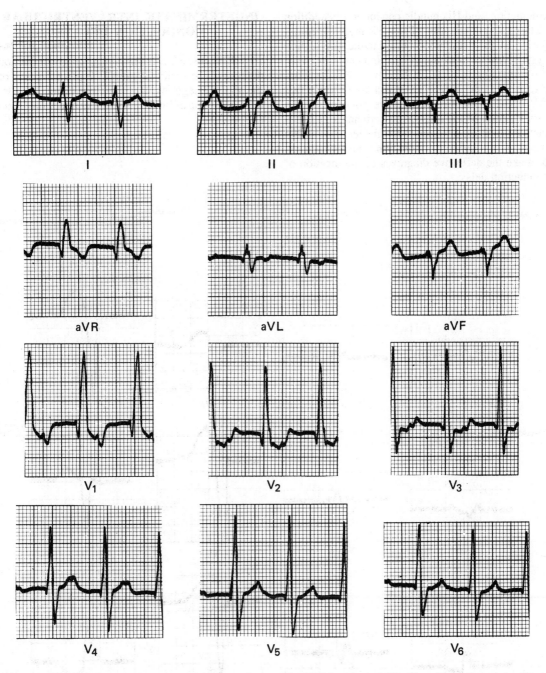

**Figure 8–18.** Possible trifascicular conduction system disease. The QRS duration is 0.13 s. The wide S waves in lead I and wide R' waves in $V_{1-2}$ are indicative of conduction delay in the right bundle branch. The initial 0.06-s frontal plane vector is −60 degrees, indicating conduction delay in the left anterior fascicle of the left bundle branch. The q waves in $V_{1-3}$ are probably too wide to be due to the anterior fascicular block and likely represent past myocardial infarction. The PR interval is 0.35 s, indicating first-degree AV block. The conduction delay resulting in the prolonged PR interval could be in the AV node or in the posterior fascicle of the left bundle branch; His bundle electrography is required for precise localization.

conduction, and His bundle conduction in addition to fascicular conduction. Thus, PR interval prolongation in the presence of bifascicular conduction system disease does not always indicate disease in the remaining fascicle of the intraventricular conduction system; in fact, there is a 50% chance that AV nodal conduction delay is responsible for the prolongation of PR interval in patients with bifascicular block. Specialized recording techniques that measure His-Purkinje conduction time are required to make the definitive diagnosis of the location of conduction delay.

## INDETERMINATE INTRAVENTRICULAR CONDUCTION DELAYS

At times, a bizarre intraventricular conduction defect will be seen that cannot be placed in any of the above categories. It is therefore called an indeterminate type of intraventricular conduction defect (Fig 8–19).

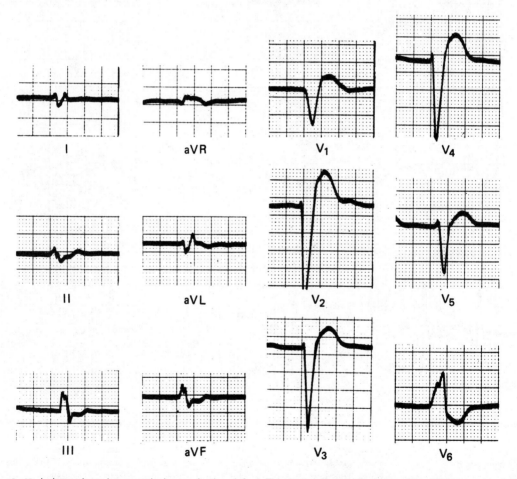

**Figure 8–19.** Indeterminate intraventricular conduction defect. The rhythm is atrial fibrillation. The QRS interval = 0.18 s. The pattern in the precordial leads is typical of left bundle branch block. A significant s wave is seen in lead I, indicating rightward forces. These findings could be the result of a greater degree of conduction delay in the left posterior fascicle than in the left anterior fascicle or could indicate associated right ventricular hypertrophy or myocardial infarction.

## TEST TRACINGS

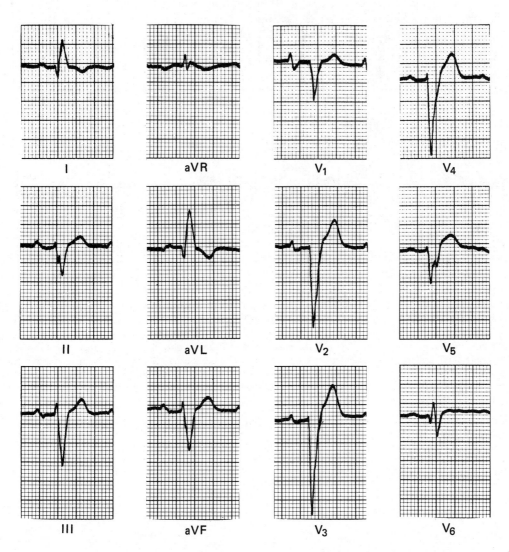

**Figure 8–T1.** Intraventricular conduction delay, superior axis deviation, and anterior wall myocardial infarction. The rhythm is sinus, the PR interval is 0.23 s, and the QRS duration is 0.15 s. The mean frontal plane QRS axis is −60 degrees, indicating left anterior fascicular block. There are wide q waves in leads I, aVL, and $V_6$ and tiny r waves in $V_{1-5}$, without significant progression in r wave voltage across the precordial leads. There is ST depression and T wave inversion in leads I and aVL and ST segment elevation in $V_{2-5}$. This ECG is consistent with left ventricular conduction delay, additional conduction delay in the region of the left anterior fascicular radiation, and septal or anterior wall myocardial infarction. It is also compatible with anterior wall myocardial infarction with peri-infarction block (conduction delay around the area of infarction, which does not involve the bundle branches themselves), and additional left anterior fascicular block. The sequential development of the electrocardiographic pattern recorded here would be required for correct interpretation.

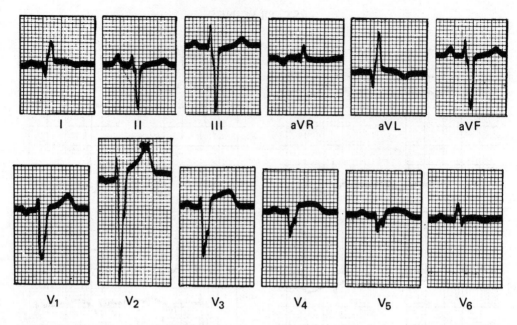

**Figure 8–T2.** Left intraventricular conduction delay and anterior wall myocardial infarction. The rhythm is sinus, the PR interval is 0.20 s, and the QRS duration is 0.12 s. The mean frontal plane QRS axis is −60 degrees, indicating left anterior fascicular conduction delay. Abnormal Q waves are present in leads I and aVL; QS complexes are present in $V_{4-5}$. ST segment elevation is seen in I, aVL, and $V_{2-6}$. The Q waves and ST segment elevation in leads $V_{4-5}$ indicate anterior wall myocardial infarction. Left anterior fascicular block alone is not expected to cause Q waves of this magnitude or duration. The left axis deviation is, however, due to anterior fascicular conduction delay. The prolongation of the QRS duration is due to an intraventricular conduction delay related to the myocardial infarction, as left anterior fascicular block does not itself prolong the intraventricular conduction time.

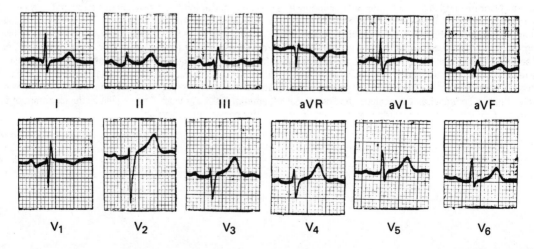

**Figure 8–T3.** Minor right-sided intraventricular conduction delay in a normal individual. The mean frontal plane QRS axis is normal. The QRS duration is 0.10 s. An rSR' complex is present in $V_1$ and aVF. The ST–T waves are normal.

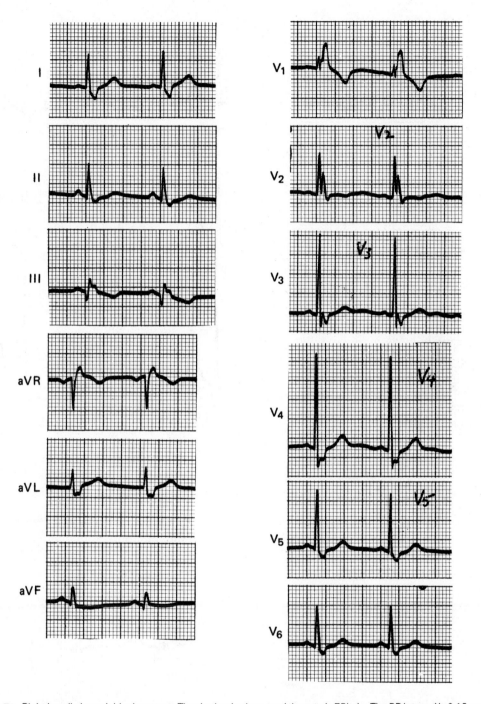

**Figure 8 –T4.** Right bundle branch block pattern. The rhythm is sinus, and the rate is 75/min. The PR interval is 0.16 s, and the QRS duration is 0.14 s. There are wide S waves in leads I and V$_{4-6}$ and a wide R' wave in lead V$_1$, indicating conduction delay in the right bundle branch. The voltage of the R' wave in V$_1$ is variable and reflects the magnitude of the conduction delay rather than hypertrophy of the underlying myocardium. Therefore, the diagnosis of right ventricular hypertrophy cannot be made on the basis of voltage of the R' wave alone; rightward deviation of the electrical axis and a qR or pure R wave in V$_1$ would be required.

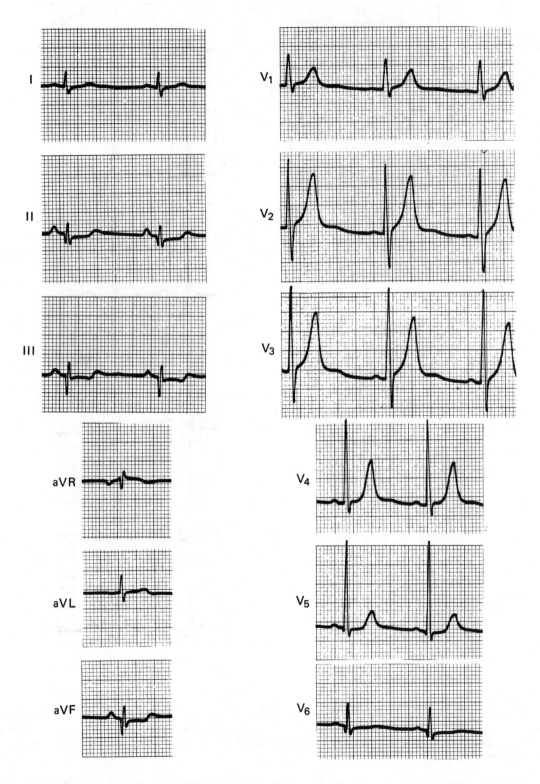

**Figure 8–T5.** Inferoposterior wall myocardial infarction (see Chapter 10). The mean frontal plane QRS axis is deviated superiorly, but this is due to loss of inferior forces, as indicated by the Q waves in leads II, III, and aVF, rather than to left anterior fascicular conduction delay. There is an abnormally tall R wave in $V_1$, but this is the result of loss of posterior forces rather than conduction delay. The QRS duration is normal, and criteria for right ventricular conduction delay (wide S wave in leads I, aVL, and $V_6$; rSR′ in $V_1$) are not met.

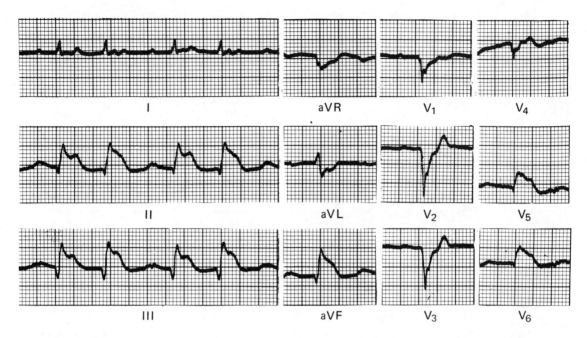

**Figure 8 – T6.** Acute inferolateral wall myocardial infarction with type I second-degree (Wenckebach) AV block (see Chapter 12). There are q waves in leads II, III, and aVF. The QS waves in $V_{1-4}$ are due to a prior anterior myocardial infarction. The ST segments are markedly elevated in II, III, aVF, and $V_{5-6}$. The ST segments should not be confused with portions of the QRS complexes, leading to the erroneous diagnosis of intraventricular conduction delay. There is ST segment depression in leads aVL and $V_{1-2}$, which could be reciprocal to the posterior infarction or indicate ischemia in these areas (see Chapter 10).

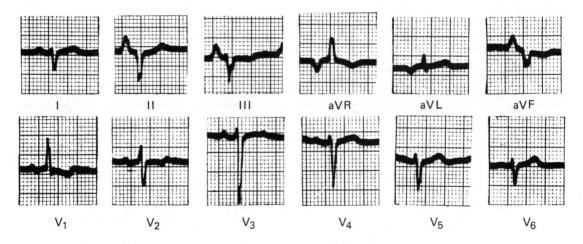

**Figure 8 – T7.** Right ventricular hypertrophy in a patient with obstructive lung disease. The rhythm is sinus, and the PR interval is 0.16 s. The QRS duration is normal at 0.08 s. The mean frontal plane QRS axis is abnormally rightward and superiorly directed, compatible with the clinical diagnosis. Right bundle branch "block" is not expected to result in deviation of the electrical axis. Although there are S waves in lead I and $V_{5-6}$, they are not broad. The R wave in $V_1$ is abnormally tall, but it is a pure R wave (and not an rSR' complex) and is not abnormally wide. The QS waves in the inferior leads do not necessarily indicate inferior wall myocardial infarction in patients with chronic obstructive pulmonary disease; the normal T waves in these leads suggest that infarction had not occurred. (At autopsy, marked right atrial and ventricular hypertrophy, without infarction, were found.)

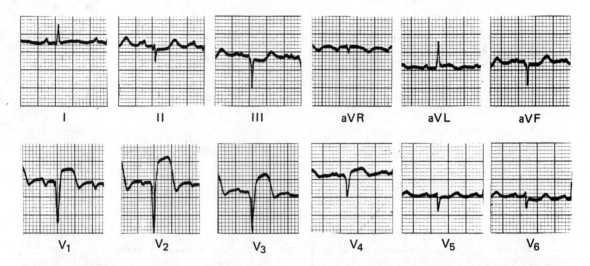

**Figure 8 –T8.** Anterior infarction with left anterior fascicular block. QS complexes with ST segment elevation and T wave inversion are present in $V_{1-4}$. These findings are evidence of acute anterior wall infarction (see Chapter 10). The mean frontal plane QRS axis is −45 degrees, indicating left anterior fascicular block.

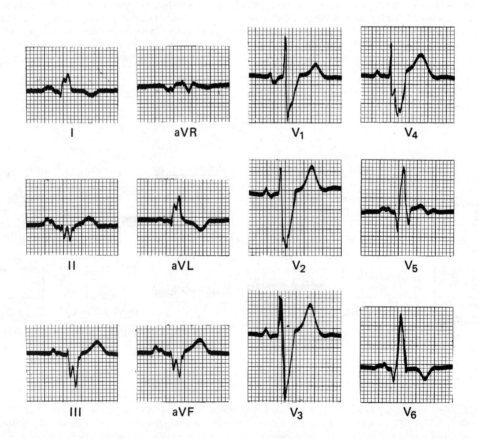

**Figure 8 –T9.** Conduction delay in the left bundle branch (with septal myocardial infarction) or anterior wall myocardial infarction with peri-infarction block. The rhythm is sinus, the PR interval is 0.16 s, the QRS duration is 0.17 s, and the mean frontal plane QRS axis is −45 degrees. The R waves are wide and notched in leads I, aVL, and $V_{5-6}$. Initial q waves are present in these leads. The presence of the q wave suggests that either the interventricular septum has been infarcted or that conduction delay around the area of infarction is present. Knowledge of the electrocardiographic pattern in prior tracings would be helpful in arriving at the proper diagnosis.

Myocardial ischemia occurs when coronary artery blood flow is insufficient to meet myocardial metabolic requirements. By definition, it is a transient and reversible phenomenon. The electrocardiographic findings usually consist of only ST segment and T wave abnormalities. Since the underlying process is transient, so are the electrocardiographic features; thus, a single ECG is never diagnostic of myocardial ischemia, since the transient, reversible nature of the abnormalities cannot be demonstrated in a single tracing. Similarly, separate ECGs recorded weeks, months, or years apart that show identical ST and T wave abnormalities are extremely unlikely to be reflecting myocardial ischemia, as ischemia is a dynamic process not expected to remain the same over time. The diagnosis of myocardial ischemia, therefore, depends upon the clinical evaluation of the patient and the electrocardiographic changes during *and after* spontaneous angina pectoris, whether it occurs at rest or during exercise. Many conditions unrelated to myocardial ischemia can produce ST and T wave abnormalities similar to those due to ischemia, including hypokalemia, left ventricular hypertrophy, drug effects, pericarditis, and myocarditis. Most commonly, however, the ST and T wave abnormalities have no clear cause and are thus idiopathic. Unless the diagnosis of myocardial ischemia is proved, the ST–T wave changes must be considered to be *nonspecific* or *nondiagnostic* and interpreted as such.

## MECHANISM OF ELECTROCARDIOGRAPHIC PATTERNS IN MYOCARDIAL ISCHEMIA

### ST Segment Changes

It is believed that currents of injury generated by the resting and active muscle produce the ST segment deviation seen in myocardial ischemia.

### Injury Current of Rest

Injured muscle is electrically negative in relation to normal resting muscle (Fig 9–1). An electrode overlying the injured area will record a depression relative to the baseline. When the muscle is stimulated, an advancing negative charge (in front of which is a positive charge) is initiated, and the overlying electrode records a positive deflection. When a potential difference no longer exists between the advancing stimulus and the injured area, the recorded deflection returns to the baseline.

When an electrode overlies an uninjured area of the muscle, the reverse occurs. As the electrode is facing a positive charge, the deflection it produces is elevated relative to the baseline (Fig 9–1). When the muscle is stimulated, a negative charge results, producing a downward deflection. When a potential difference between the uninjured and the injured areas of the muscle is not present, the deflection returns to the baseline. Since the original deflection was elevated relative to the baseline, the inscribed deflection gives the appearance of ST segment depression. When the muscle returns to its resting state, the deflection returns to its resting position (Fig 9–1).

### Injury Current of Activity

Experimental evidence suggests that when injured muscle is stimulated, it does not become as electrically negative as normal muscle. Thus, stimulated injured muscle will have less of a negative charge and therefore a larger positive charge than normal stimulated muscle. An electrode overlying the injured portion of a muscle will face this positive charge, resulting in elevation of the ST segment (Fig 9–2). An electrode overlying the uninjured portion of the muscle will face a negative charge, resulting in depression of the ST segment. As a practical rule, an electrocardiographic tracing recorded directly over injured muscle records ST segment elevation. If normal muscle lies between injured muscle and the recording electrode, ST segment depression results (Fig 9–3).

### T Wave Changes

As a result of the ST segment depression, the T wave may be "dragged" downward, producing the appearance of T wave inversion; however, true T

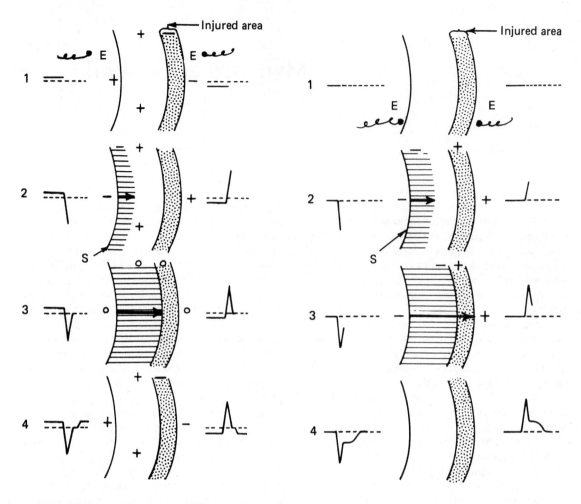

**Figure 9–1.** Injury current of rest. (The dotted lines indicate the isoelectric baseline.) The injured area is negative relative to the rest of the muscle. (1) An electrode (E) overlying the injured muscle will record a depression relative to the baseline, and an electrode overlying the noninjured muscle will record an elevation relative to the baseline. When the muscle is stimulated (S) (2), an advancing negative charge (in front of which is a positive charge) exists, producing an upward deflection recorded by the electrode overlying the injured area and a downward deflection recorded by the electrode overlying the noninjured area. When there ceases to be a potential difference between the injured and uninjured areas of the muscle, the deflections return to the baseline (3). When the muscle returns to its resting state, the deflections recorded from the 2 electrodes return to their original positions (4); the electrode overlying the injured area records ST segment elevation, and the electrode overlying the noninjured area records ST segment depression.

**Figure 9–2.** Injury current of activity.

wave inversion also occurs in leads showing ST segment depression (Fig 9–4).

## ELECTROCARDIOGRAPHIC PATTERNS RESULTING FROM MYOCARDIAL ISCHEMIA

### ST Segment Depression

ST segment depression reflects **nontransmural myocardial ischemia.** It often involves the subendocardial areas of the heart, which are the most vulnerable to ischemic injury due both to their bearing the brunt of systolic pressure developed by the ventricle and their smaller total blood supply. The typical electrocardiographic pattern is ST segment depression with T wave inversion in left ventricular epicardial leads (Fig 9–4) and ST segment elevation (often not discernible) in leads facing the nonischemic portion of ventricular tissue.

Occasionally, the T waves may be abnormal in a baseline tracing recorded in a patient with angina

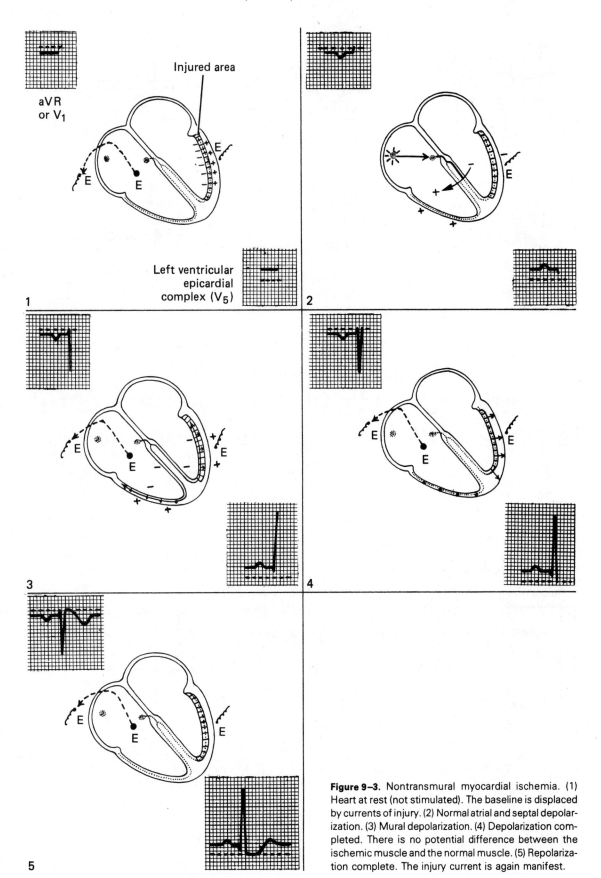

aVR
or V₁

Injured area

Left ventricular
epicardial
complex (V₅)

1

2

3

4

5

**Figure 9–3.** Nontransmural myocardial ischemia. (1) Heart at rest (not stimulated). The baseline is displaced by currents of injury. (2) Normal atrial and septal depolarization. (3) Mural depolarization. (4) Depolarization completed. There is no potential difference between the ischemic muscle and the normal muscle. (5) Repolarization complete. The injury current is again manifest.

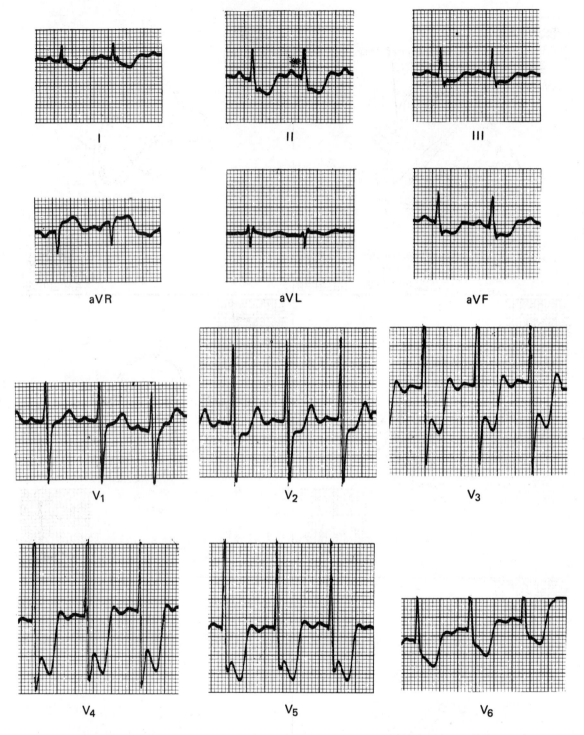

**Figure 9–4.** Marked, diffuse ST segment depression with T wave inversion recorded in a patient with 3-vessel coronary artery disease during an episode of anginal pain. Tracings before and after the pain were entirely normal. ST segment depression is most prominent in II, III, aVF, and V$_{2-6}$; in leads V$_{3-5}$ the ST depression is 10 mm.

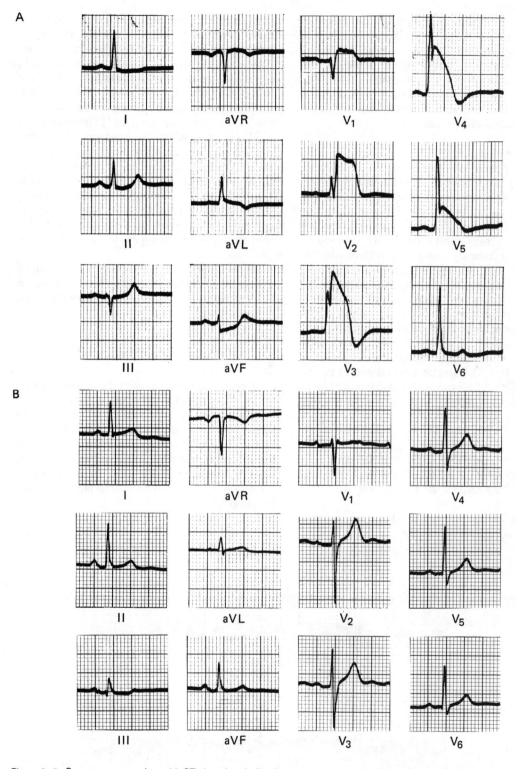

**Figure 9–5.** Spontaneous angina with ST elevation, indicating transmural myocardial ischemia. *A:* Tracing taken during an episode of anginal pain that occurred while the patient was at bed rest in the hospital. There is marked ST elevation in leads $V_{2-5}$ with ST depression in aVF. *B:* Tracing taken 30 min after (A) when the patient was pain-free and asymptomatic. The ST segments are isoelectric, and the ECG is normal. Subsequent evaluation, including serial ECGs and enzyme determinations, revealed no evidence of acute myocardial infarction. Although tracing (A) is quite typical of early infarction (see Chapter 10), the rapid disappearance of the ST elevation and the absence of clinical and electrocardiographic evidence of infarction on subsequent examinations indicate that tracing (A) represents severe acute but reversible ischemia.

pectoris. During pain, these T waves may become upright ("normalization"). This phenomenon is termed "pseudonormalization" of baseline abnormal T waves and, in the presence of acute cardiac pain, indicates myocardial ischemia. However, since pseudonormalization of T waves may occur in conditions other than acute ischemia, this diagnosis requires clinical correlation.

### ST Segment Elevation

ST segment elevation (Fig 9–5) reflects **transmural myocardial ischemia** and therefore indicates a more severe degree of ischemia than is responsible for the pattern of ST segment depression. Transient reversible transmural myocardial ischemia occurring at rest is frequently observed in patients with coronary vasospasm, with or without underlying fixed obstructive coronary artery disease. If ST segment elevation develops during exercise, it may reflect vasospasm or a critical degree of coronary artery luminal obstruction, provided Q waves of prior myocardial infarction are not present. ST segment depression is often observed in leads opposite to those recording the ST segment elevation. This ST segment depression may be reciprocal to the ST elevation (Fig 9–5) or may indicate additional ischemia in areas remote from those showing ST elevation.

### PSEUDODEPRESSION & PSEUDO-ELEVATION VERSUS ISCHEMIC DEPRESSION & ELEVATION

Some normal individuals show apparent ST segment depression or elevation either at rest or during exercise. This phenomenon is usually associated with tachycardia or anxiety and is explained by the presence of a prominent atrial repolarization ($T_a$) wave. In pseudodepression, the $T_a$ wave is seen through ventricular depolarization and is still evident after the inscription of the QRS complex. This pattern can be distinguished from ischemic ST segment depression by (1) the contour of the ST segment, which in pseudodepression displays a continuous ascent with upward concavity; and (2) associated downsloping of the PR segment. In ischemic ST segment depression, the ST segment is horizontal or downsloping (or very slowly upsloping). In pseudoelevation, the $T_a$ wave may appear to represent isoelectricity, and the subsequent ST segment may therefore appear to be elevated (Fig 9–6).

In addition to $T_a$ waves, superimposition of atrial flutter waves upon the terminal portions of the QRS complexes can cause pseudodepression and pseudoelevation.

### INVERTED U WAVES

Occasionally, inversion of the U wave may be seen on a resting ECG or, more commonly, after exercise (Fig 9–7). This finding is considered to represent severe obstructive coronary artery disease involving the left anterior descending coronary artery; it is an insensitive marker for this condition, however, and its specificity is not known. An inverted U wave may also be seen in left ventricular hypertrophy.

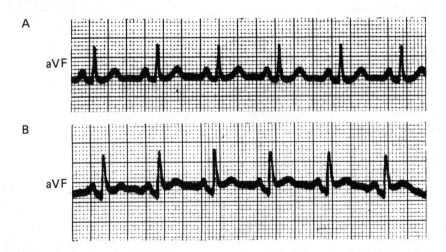

**Figure 9–6.** Pseudo-ST elevation. *A:* Normal tracing. *B:* Although the ST segment appears to be elevated, it is in fact isoelectric and on the same level as the TP segment. The downsloping PR segment, caused by a prominent $T_a$ wave, causes the apparent ST segment elevation.

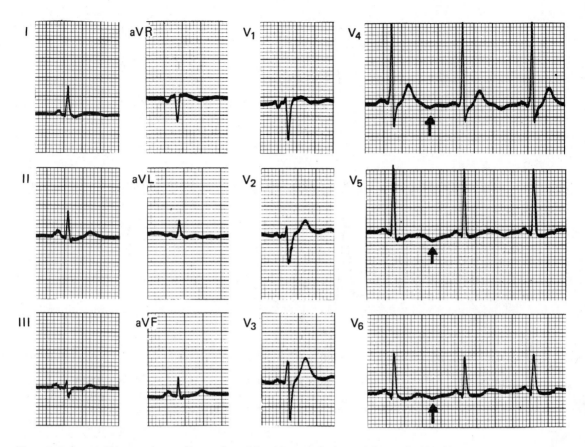

**Figure 9–7.** Inverted U waves (arrows) in a patient with aortic regurgitation and chest pain. Mild ST depression is present in I, II, aVL, and V₄₋₆. Inverted U waves are best seen in V₄₋₆.

## PROVOCATION OF MYOCARDIAL ISCHEMIA BY EXERCISE TESTING

Since the resting ECG is normal in 25–40% of patients with angina, exercise tests have been developed to provoke myocardial ischemia. Exercise test protocols are designed to impose incremental work loads on the patient, with a resulting increase in heart rate and blood pressure. The product of heart rate and systolic blood pressure (the **double product**) is an index of myocardial oxygen consumption; the exercise-induced increase in double product should be met by an increase in myocardial blood flow, unless this is limited by obstructive coronary artery disease or spasm. If coronary blood flow is insufficient to meet the metabolic demands of the myocardium, myocardial ischemia develops, with its attendant effects on the ECG. ST segment and T wave abnormalities indicative of myocardial ischemia are as follows: ST segment elevation, which reflects transmural injury (in the absence of past myocardial infarction), and ST segment depression, which reflects nontransmural injury. ST segment depression is further characterized as downsloping, horizontal, and slowly upsloping (Fig

9–8); in all cases, the J point must be depressed at least 1 mm below the isoelectric baseline for the diagnosis of myocardial ischemia to be considered. (J point depression with a rapidly upsloping ST segment is a normal response to exercise.)

Downsloping ST depression is the most specific electrocardiographic abnormality for the diagnosis of coronary artery disease based on the coronary arteriogram (exceeding 95%) and usually indicates severe multivessel disease. Horizontal ST depression is slightly less specific (85%), followed by slowly upsloping ST depression —at least 2 mm below the baseline 80 ms after the J point (75–80%). ST segment elevation indicates severe occlusive disease or coronary spasm.

Certain conditions and medications can produce ST segment and T wave abnormalities that mimic myocardial ischemia (Table 9–1); thus, the electrocardiographic response to exercise in these patients cannot be interpreted as indicating ischemia due to coronary artery disease (this is termed a "false-positive" exercise test response), although ischemia may in fact be present on grounds other than coronary disease.

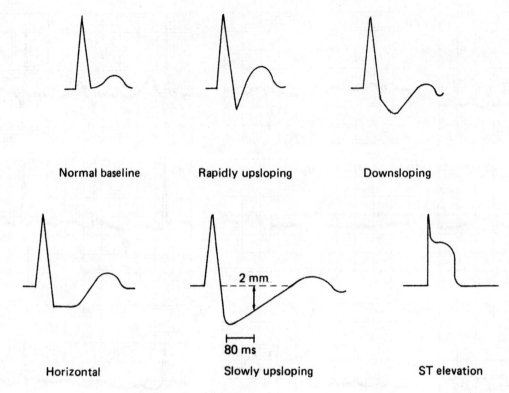

**Figure 9–8.** Types of ST segment responses to exercise.

**Table 9–1.** Causes of "false-positive" exercise electrocardiographic responses.

(1) Hyperventilation
(2) Abnormalities of left ventricular depolarization and repolarization
    Left ventricular hypertrophy
    Left bundle branch block
    Wolff-Parkinson-White conduction (see Chapter 16)
(3) Digitalis administration
(4) Vasoregulatory abnormalities
(5) Mitral valve prolapse
(6) Female sex

Myocardial infarction occurs when insufficient coronary artery blood flow causes death of myocardial tissue. This may result from atherosclerotic obstruction in the coronary arteries, thrombotic or embolic occlusion of a coronary artery, or spasm in an artery. The left ventricle is involved in virtually all instances of myocardial infarction; isolated right ventricular myocardial infarction is extremely rare. A single ECG recorded during acute myocardial infarction may be normal, may show nondiagnostic ST and T wave abnormalities only, or may reflect transmural ischemia and loss of ventricular forces. Serial ECGs and clinical correlation are mandatory in making the correct diagnosis.

It has recently become clear that the description of myocardial infarction as "nontransmural" ("subendocardial") and "transmural" is an oversimplification and therefore not correct. Electrocardiographic patterns of myocardial infarction that do not show Q waves (the classic criteria for transmural myocardial infarction) are often shown at autopsy to have been associated with necrosis of the entire ventricular myocardium from endocardium to epicardium. Conversely, ECGs that do show Q waves suggesting transmural infarction may be found at autopsy to have been limited to one or more layers of myocardium. Thus, the electrocardiographic distinction between transmural and nontransmural infarction based on the presence of Q waves is misleading. In recognition of this lack of specificity of the ECG for the anatomic situation, myocardial infarction will be described in this section as either transmural or nontransmural.

## MECHANISM OF THE ELECTROCARDIOGRAPHIC PATTERNS

### The Abnormal Q Wave & QS Complex in Transmural Infarction

The most diagnostic electrocardiographic finding for myocardial infarction is the inscription of an abnormally wide (0.04 s) and deep (25% of the height of the R wave in a given lead) q wave or QS complex. Small, nonpathologic q waves that do not meet these criteria for width and depth are seen in normal individuals, where they are commonly recorded in leads I, aVF, and $V_{4-6}$ and represent left-to-right depolarization of the interventricular septum. These nonpathologic q waves should not exceed 0.02 s or 25% of the height of the R wave.

There are 3 exceptions to the criteria given above for the diagnosis of a pathologic Q wave: (1) If the Q wave is confined to lead III, it has no special significance. Q waves 0.04 s in duration and 25% of the height of the R wave may be recorded in normal individuals whose mean frontal plane QRS axis lies between +30 and 0 degrees; lead aVF will not record a q wave. Thus, the diagnosis of myocardial infarction based on the presence of Q waves isolated to lead III should not be made. (2) If the q wave is confined to lead aVL alone and there are no other abnormalities in the ECG, it has no special significance. Q waves 0.04 s in duration and 25% of the height of the R wave may be recorded in normal persons whose mean frontal plane QRS axis is vertical (between +60 and +90 degrees). (3) A small q wave (but not a QR or QS complex) may be present in lead $V_2$. While any q wave in this lead is often an abnormal finding, it may indicate conditions other than myocardial infarction (such as left bundle branch block, left anterior fascicular block, left ventricular hypertrophy, or chronic obstructive pulmonary disease) and thus is not helpful in establishing the diagnosis of infarction.

The genesis of the Q wave is the redirection of electrical forces due to loss of forces. An electrocardiographic recording at a given moment in time represents the mean of electrical forces going in many directions in space. Ninety percent of such forces are canceled, leaving only about 10% that are recorded. When a myocardial infarction of significant size occurs, the depolarization forces in that area are lost, resulting in a change of direction of mean forces away from the area of infarction (Fig 10–1). The redirection of forces occurs most significantly during the initial 0.04-0.05 s of ventricular depolarization, resulting in a q wave (or QR or QS complex) in leads overlying the infarction zone. A small infarction, in which only a small amount of

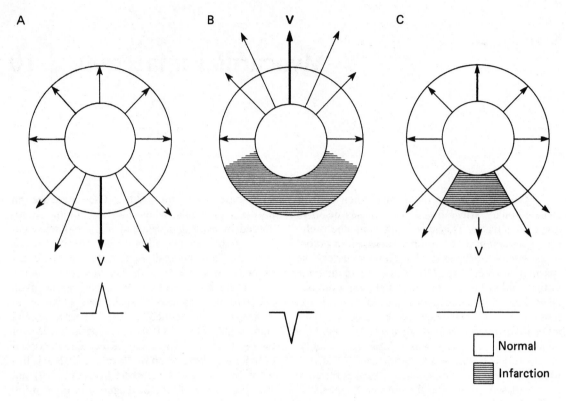

**Figure 10–1.** Cross section of the ventricle, showing arrows directed from the endocardium to the epicardium, representing the first 0.04 s of ventricular depolarization. *A:* Normal myocardium, in which there are greater forces directed downward, resulting in a mean force in that direction (heavy arrow) and an upright complex recorded by an electrode overlying that area. *B:* Loss of large forces because of myocardial necrosis, resulting in the mean force now being oriented in an opposite direction (heavy arrow). The electrode overlying the area of necrosis records a negative deflection (Q wave). *C:* Loss of some forces because of a small amount of myocardial necrosis, resulting in a reduction of mean force directed downward. The electrode overlying this area may not record a q wave but only a small R wave.

tissue is lost, may be insufficient to alter the mean forces so as to produce a q wave but may merely reduce the magnitude of the normal mean force, resulting in a reduction in R wave voltage in the leads overlying the infarction zone. It should be emphasized that a *reduction* in R wave voltage across the precordium (rather than lack of the expected *progression* of R wave voltage) may be an indicator of infarction, provided that other electrocardiographic abnormalities (such as ST and T wave changes) are also present.

## ST Segment Changes in Transmural Infarction

Frequently, the first electrocardiographic finding in myocardial infarction is ST segment elevation in a lead overlying the area of infarction. The ST segment characteristically has a convex upward curvature.

Leads that are placed approximately 180 degrees from the area of infarction show reciprocal ST segment depression. These changes are analogous to those described for injury currents in the isolated muscle strip.

It should be appreciated that ST segment depression might also reflect additional ischemia in the area of myocardium recorded by those ECG leads; thus, the differential diagnosis between *reciprocal* ST segment depression and ischemia remote from the area of infarction often must be made by independent means.

Because completely dead muscle is believed not to produce ST segment changes, the occurrence of these changes early in infarction indicates the presence of some viable muscle in the epicardial region.

## T Wave Changes in Transmural Infarction

Within the first few hours of infarction, "giant" upright T waves may be seen in leads overlying the infarct. The exact cause is not known but may be leakage of intracellular potassium from the damaged muscle cells into the extracellular spaces.

After a period of hours or days (up to 2 weeks), the ST segment returns to the isoelectric line and T wave changes occur. The T wave changes may begin to develop while the ST segments are still deviated. The T waves begin to invert in those leads that showed ST segment elevation.

The typical infarction T wave is inverted and symmetric; that is, its peak is midway between the beginning and the end. The inverted T wave may have an isoelectric ST segment but show an upward convexity ("coronary" T wave), or it may have an elevated ST segment and an upward convexity ("cove-plane" T wave).

In transmural infarctions, the abnormal Q waves may appear within hours of infarction or much later in its evolution. They may occur while the ST segment changes are present or appear after they have become isoelectric. Q waves usually appear before marked T wave changes have occurred.

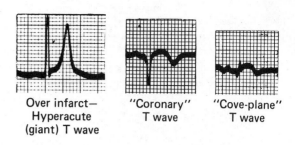

Over infarct— Hyperacute (giant) T wave     "Coronary" T wave     "Cove-plane" T wave

## LOCALIZATION OF TRANSMURAL INFARCTION BY ELECTROCARDIOGRAPHIC PATTERNS

By observing the infarction pattern in specific electrocardiographic leads, the anatomic site of infarction can often be localized.

The blood supply to the heart is derived from the left and right coronary arteries, which arise from the left and right aortic sinuses, respectively. Shortly after its origin, the left coronary artery divides into the left anterior descending and the left

circumflex arteries (Fig 10–2). The former supplies the anterior surface of the left ventricle, the medial portion of the anterior surface of the right ventricle, and the lower third of the posterior surface of the right ventricle. The remainder of the right ventricle is supplied by the right coronary artery. The circumflex artery supplies the lateral wall and the lower (apical) half of the posterior wall of the left ventricle. The upper (basal) half of the posterior wall and the inferior wall of the left ventricle are supplied by the right coronary artery. Anatomic variations exist, depending upon the "dominance" of the right and left coronary systems. In atherosclerotic and vasospastic coronary disease, the blood supply to different areas of the myocardium will vary, depending upon the site and magnitude of the arterial obstruction and the presence and integrity of the collateral circulation.

The site of infarction can be determined by

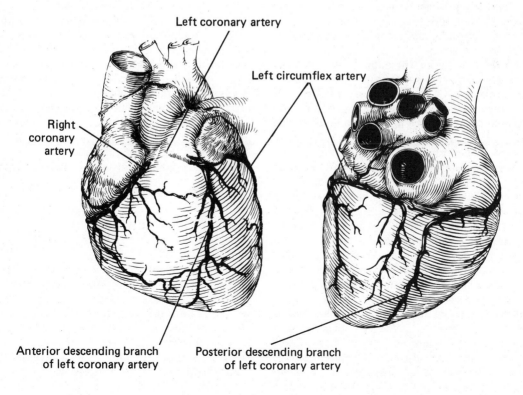

Left coronary artery

Left circumflex artery

Right coronary artery

Anterior descending branch of left coronary artery

Posterior descending branch of left coronary artery

**Figure 10–2.** Coronary circulation.

applying the electrocardiographic criteria for diagnosis of myocardial infarction to specific leads.

| Site of Infarction | Electrocardiographic Leads Reflecting the Infarction |
|---|---|
| Anterior | $V_{2-6}$ |
| Inferior | II and aVF (and III) |
| Lateral | I, aVL, and $V_6$ |
| Posterior | $V_{1-2}$ |
| Right ventricle | $V_{2-4R}$ |

## ANTERIOR WALL MYOCARDIAL INFARCTION

Anterior wall myocardial infarction is best reflected in the precordial leads. Leads I and aVL may show the infarction pattern if lateral wall myocardial infarction is also present. The characteristic findings in the evolution of a transmural anterior wall myocardial infarction are summarized as follows (Fig 10–3):

**Frontal plane:** ST segment elevation occurs in leads I and aVL, reflecting transmural injury, followed by the inscription of a Q wave, reflecting loss of myocardium, and, finally, T wave inversion. Leads II and III may show ST segment depression, which is either reciprocal to the ST elevation or reflective of additional ischemia remote from the area of infarction.

**Precordial leads:** Depending upon the extent of the infarction and the position of the heart within the chest, several of the precordial leads will show the infarction pattern.

**Vector analysis:** The initial 0.04-s vector is directed posteriorly, away from the infarction zone, resulting in a q or QS wave in the precordial leads. If this initial vector is also oriented rightward, an abnormal q wave will be inscribed in lead I. In the early stages of myocardial infarction, the ST vector is oriented anteriorly and to the left, resulting in ST segment elevation in lead I and the left precordial leads. Within the first few hours of infarction, tall ("giant"), tented T waves may be recorded in the leads overlying the infarcted area. The tented T waves are thought to reflect local hyperkalemia due to potassium efflux from necrotic tissue. In later stages, the T vector is oriented posteriorly and to the right, producing inverted T waves in these leads.

When a pattern of infarction involving the *inferior* leads occurs in association with an *anterior* wall myocardial infarction, it is likely that there is only a single infarction, involving both the anterior wall and the apical area of the heart. Leads II and aVF (and sometimes also III) may therefore show the infarction pattern, as they reflect events occurring at the cardiac apex (Fig 10–4). However, the possibility does exist that both anterior and inferior

wall myocardial infarction may occur at the same time (Fig 10–5).

## INFERIOR WALL MYOCARDIAL INFARCTION

Since this area of myocardium overlies the left diaphragm, the infarction pattern will be recorded in leads II, III, and aVF. The characteristic findings of transmural infarction in this area are summarized as follows (Fig 10–6):

**Frontal plane:** The infarct pattern will be seen in leads II, III, and aVF. At the time of ST segment elevation in these leads, reciprocal ST segment depression may be seen in leads I and aVL. Later, when the T waves become inverted in the inferior leads, the T waves in leads I and aVL will become tall.

**Precordial leads:** The precordial leads often show no abnormality. At times, however, depending upon the extent of infarction, abnormalities will be recorded in the area of the interventricular septum ($V_{2-3}$) or in the area of the lateral wall ($V_6$). Not infrequently, ST segment depression, which is either reciprocal to the ST segment elevation or indicative of anterior wall ischemia, is recorded in $V_{1-3}$.

**Vector analysis:** The initial 0.04-s vector is directed superiorly because of the loss of inferior forces. Thus, abnormal Q waves are inscribed in leads II, III, and aVF, and the mean frontal plane QRS axis is directed leftward and superiorly. It is important to recognize that the superior axis deviation in the presence of inferior wall myocardial infarction is due not to conduction system disease involving the left anterior fascicle of the left bundle branch (see Chapter 8) but to loss of muscle. In the early stage of infarction, the ST vector is directed inferiorly, producing ST segment elevation in these leads. In the later stages, the T vector is oriented superiorly, resulting in inverted T waves in II, III, and aVF.

## POSTERIOR WALL MYOCARDIAL INFARCTION

Myocardial infarction confined to the posterior wall of the heart is unusual; posterior wall infarction is almost always accompanied by inferior or lateral wall myocardial infarction (or both). In addition to the electrocardiographic pattern of inferior wall infarction, therefore, that of posterior wall infarction is added. As a result of posterior wall infarction, the initial 0.04 s of the QRS complex will be directed anteriorly, because of loss of the forces normally generated by the posterior portion of the ventricle

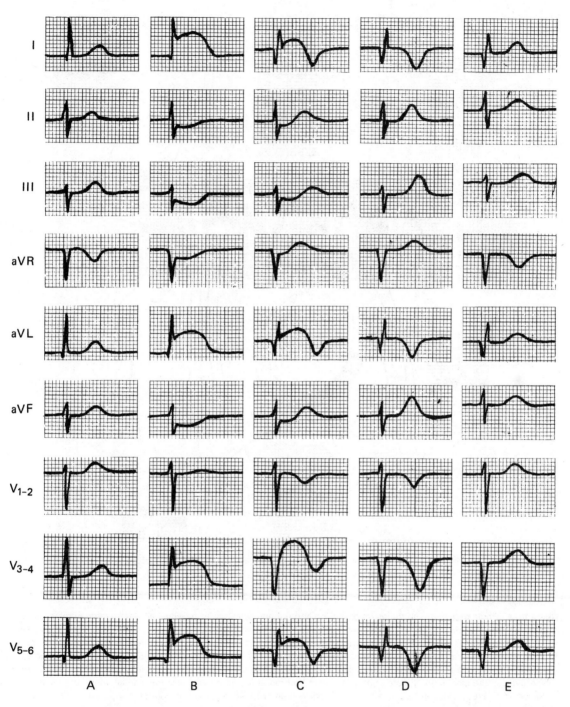

**Figure 10–3.** Diagrammatic illustration of serial electrocardiographic patterns in anterior wall myocardial infarction. **A:** Normal tracing. **B:** Early pattern. There is ST segment elevation in I, aVL, and V$_{3-6}$ and ST depression in II, III, and aVF (the ST depression might reflect inferior wall ischemia or reciprocal depression). **C:** Later pattern (hours to days). Q waves are present in I, aVL, and V$_{5-6}$. QS complexes are present in V$_{3-4}$, indicating that the major area of infarction underlies the area recorded by V$_{3-4}$. ST segment changes persist but to a lesser degree, and the T waves are beginning to invert in those leads in which ST segment elevation is present. **D:** Late (established) pattern (days to weeks). The Q waves and QS complexes persist. The ST segments are isoelectric. The T waves are deeply and symmetrically inverted in the leads that showed ST elevation and tall in the leads that showed ST depression. This pattern may persist for the remainder of the patient's life. **E:** Very late pattern (months to years). The abnormal Q waves and QS complexes persist, but the T waves have returned to normal. Without the benefit of serial ECGs, it is not possible to determine when myocardial infarction occurred. Therefore, no conclusions should be drawn as to the age of the process on the basis of a single ECG.

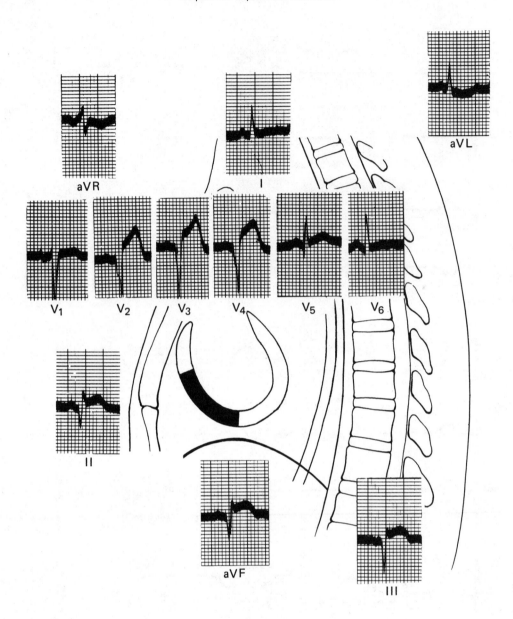

**Figure 10–4.** Single myocardial infarction involving the anterior and apical walls, in which all electrocardiographic changes occur over the same period of time. There are deep, wide Q waves with elevated ST segments in leads II and III. Lead aVF shows a Q wave and ST elevation. This pattern indicates inferior wall myocardial infarction. The precordial leads show loss of R wave voltage between $V_1$ and $V_2$, QS complexes in $V_{3-4}$ and a qR complex in $V_5$. There is ST segment elevation in $V_{2-5}$, reflecting anterior wall myocardial infarction. The abnormalities in the inferior leads reflect infarction of the cardiac apex, which overlies the diaphragm in some patients. Since both anterior and inferior wall myocardial infarctions might have occurred at different times in this patient, clinical correlation is most important in correct interpretation of the site of infarction.

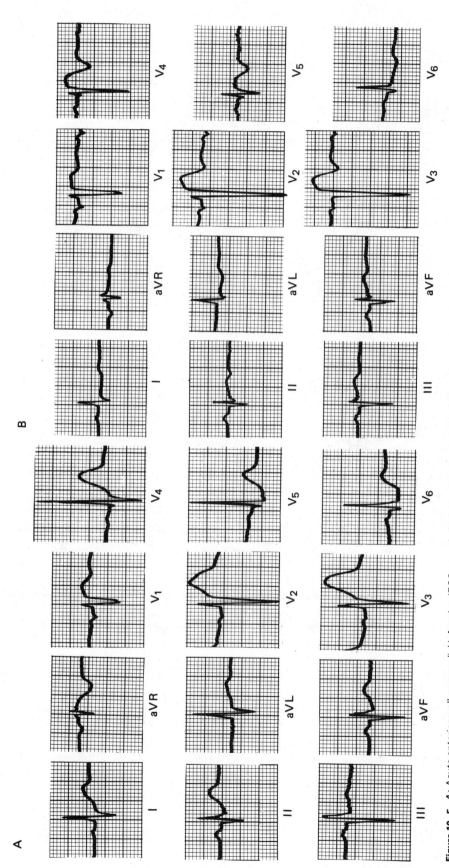

**Figure 10–5.** *A*: Acute anterior wall myocardial infarction (ECG recorded 1 hour after the onset of chest pain) and old inferior wall myocardial infarction (known to have occurred 1 year before). The anterior wall infarction is indicated by the ST elevation in $V_{1-3}$, the ST depression in $V_{5-6}$, and the large, broad, upright T waves in I, II, and $V_{2-4}$. There are QR complexes in II, III, and aVF, but the ST segments and T waves are *normal*. *B*: ECG recorded 24 hours later. The large T waves are no longer present, and there is now T wave inversion in I, aVL, and the precordial leads. A QS complex has appeared in $V_3$, and the R wave voltage has decreased in $V_{4-6}$. Thus, the *serial* changes in these ECGs have involved only the anterior wall; whereas no serial changes have occurred in the inferior leads.

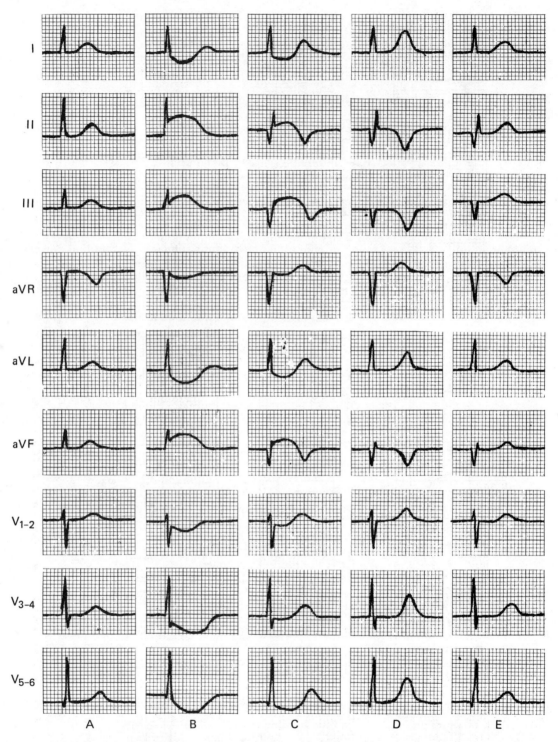

**Figure 10–6.** Diagrammatic illustration of serial electrocardiographic patterns in inferior myocardial infarction. *A:* Normal tracing. *B:* Very early pattern (hours after infarction). There is ST segment elevation in II, III, and aVF and ST segment depression in I, aVL, and aVR as well as in the precordial leads. *C:* Later pattern (hours to days). Abnormal Q waves have appeared in the inferior leads. There is less ST elevation in these leads and less ST depression in the anterior leads. The T waves are becoming inverted in II, III, and aVF. *D:* Late (established) pattern (days to weeks). The ST segments are isoelectric. Deep, symmetrically inverted T waves are seen in II, III, and aVF. The T waves are abnormally tall and symmetric in I, aVL, and the precordial leads. This pattern may persist for the remainder of the patient's life. *E:* Very late (months to years) pattern. The abnormal Q waves persist, but the T waves have become normal.

(Fig 10–7). This condition will result in abnormally tall R waves in precordial leads $V_{1-2}$. Q waves may be recorded over the posterior surface of the heart by esophageal electrodes. ST segment depression in $V_{1-2}$ is seen early in posterior wall myocardial infarction, which might be reciprocal to posterior wall ST elevation or might reflect additional anterior wall myocardial ischemia. Later, tall, symmetric T waves will be present.

## Inferoposterolateral Wall Myocardial Infarction

The pattern of infarction will be recorded in the inferior leads, the anterior precordial leads, and the lateral leads. The inferior infarction will be manifested by abnormal Q waves and T wave inversion in II, III, and aVF. The posterior wall infarction will be manifested by abnormally tall R waves with upright T waves in $V_{1-2}$. The lateral wall infarction will be manifested by abnormal Q waves and inverted T waves in $V_{5-7}$ (Fig 10–8).

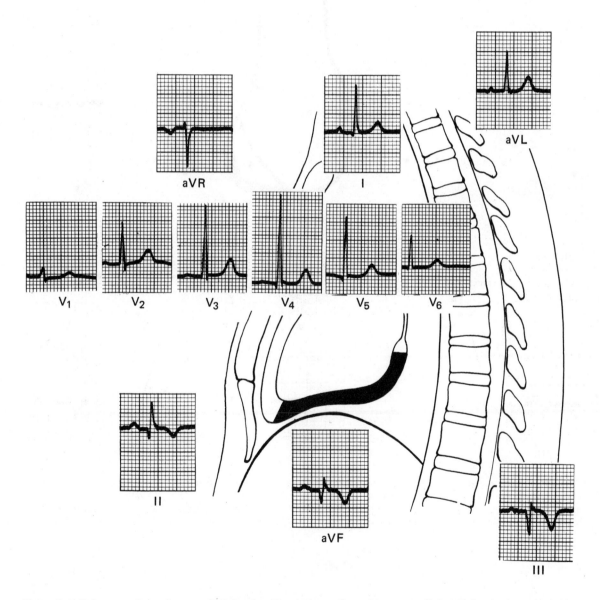

**Figure 10–7.** Inferoposterior wall myocardial infarction. The electrocardiographic pattern of inferior infarction is seen in leads II, III, and aVF. The posterior wall infarction is manifested by an abnormally tall R wave in $V_{1-2}$, indicating loss of posterior forces with consequent prominent anterior forces. The T waves are upright in $V_{1-2}$, indicating an anteriorly directed T wave vector. The tall R waves in leads $V_{1-2}$ might be due to right ventricular hypertrophy (see Chapter 7), but right axis deviation, tall, peaked P waves, and T wave inversion in $V_{1-2}$ are all absent, whereas criteria for inferior infarction are present. Thus, the diagnosis of right ventricular hypertrophy is unlikely.

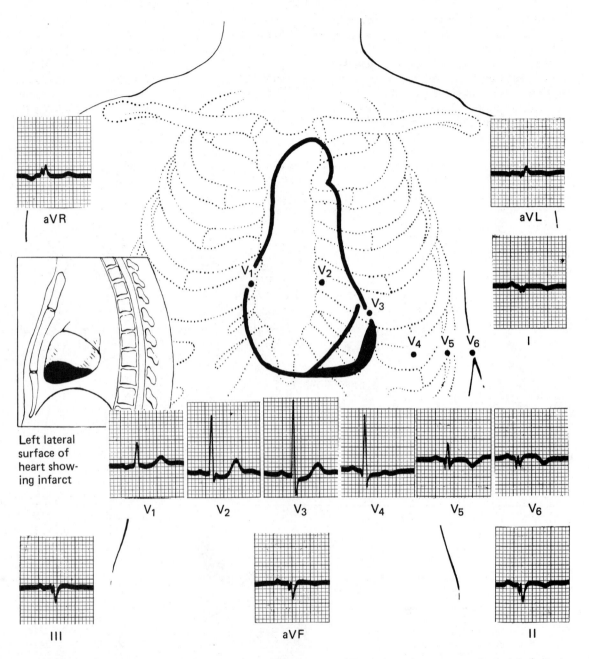

**Figure 10–8.** Inferoposterolateral wall myocardial infarction. Q waves and T wave inversion are present in the inferior leads, abnormally tall R waves with upright T waves are present in precordial leads $V_{1-2}$, and Q waves with T wave inversion are present in lateral leads $V_{5-6}$. The mean frontal plane QRS axis is directed rightward because of loss of left lateral forces. The rightward axis deviation does not reflect increased muscle mass of the right ventricle (right ventricular hypertrophy).

## NONTRANSMURAL MYOCARDIAL INFARCTION

As mentioned previously, although the ECG was used for many years to distinguish transmural from nontransmural myocardial infarction, it is now recognized that this differentiation cannot be made from the ECG alone. It had been considered that the subendocardial portion of the myocardium was electrically "silent" and that depolarization in this area would not be associated with an abnormal Q wave. However, correlations of electrocardiographic patterns with autopsy findings have clearly documented the unreliability of the ECG in establishing an accurate differential anatomic diagnosis. Although many transmural infarctions are manifested by Q waves on the ECG, a significant number are not (Fig 10–9); conversely, many nontransmural infarctions will demonstrate Q waves. When Q waves are not present, the electrocardiographic diagnosis of acute myocardial infarction depends upon evolutionary changes in serial records and clinical correlation. The differential diagnosis of nontransmural infarction from myocardial ischemia likewise depends upon the serial demonstration of evolutionary changes in the former and reversibility to normal (or baseline) in the latter; a single ECG is insufficient for the correct diagnosis.

## MULTIPLE INFARCTIONS

If the ECG reverts to normal after an initial infarction, a second infarct will produce a pattern as would be expected with initial infarction.

The abnormal Q waves which may persist following the initial infarct may not be altered by a second infarct involving the opposite wall. However, the ST segment elevations that will occur with the second infarct will cause ST segment depression in the area of the initial infarct. The development of inverted T waves as a result of the second infarct can cause the inverted T waves resulting from the initial infarct to become upright (Figs 10–10 and 10–11).

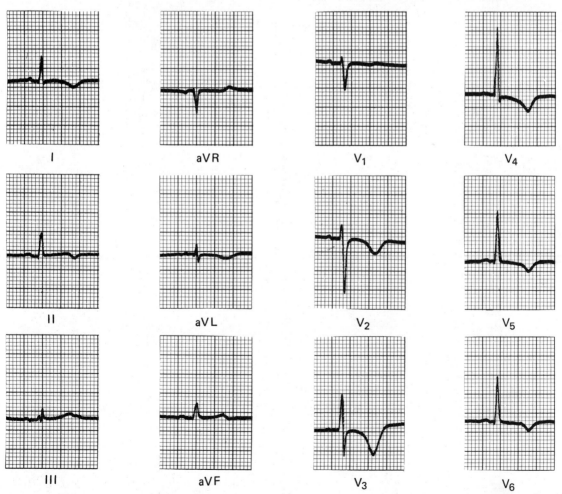

**Figure 10–9.** Nontransmural (non–Q wave) myocardial infarction, documented at autopsy to be transmural. The T waves are symmetrically inverted in I, II, aVL, and V₂₋₆. Q waves are not present, despite the through-and-through infarction process.

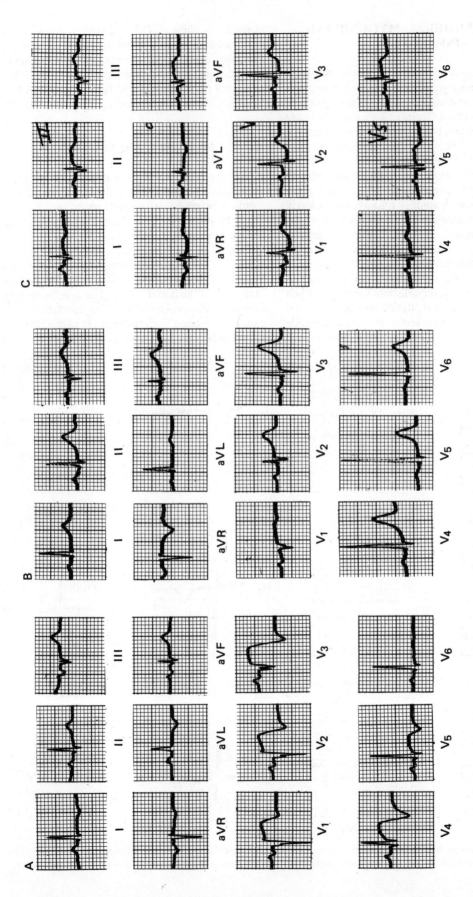

**Figure 10–10.** Multiple myocardial infarctions. *A:* Acute anterior wall myocardial infarction. Deep Q waves are present in leads $V_{1-3}$ with ST segment elevation in leads $V_{1-5}$ and T wave inversion in leads I, aVL, and $V_{1-5}$. *B:* Ten months later, the ECG has reverted to normal. *C:* Second acute myocardial infarction, occurring 8 months after the tracing in (B) was recorded. New Q waves with ST segment elevation are present in leads I, II, III, aVF, and $V_{5-6}$. Abnormally tall R waves are present in $V_{1-2}$, with ST segment depression in these leads. This second myocardial infarction is inferoposterolateral in location.

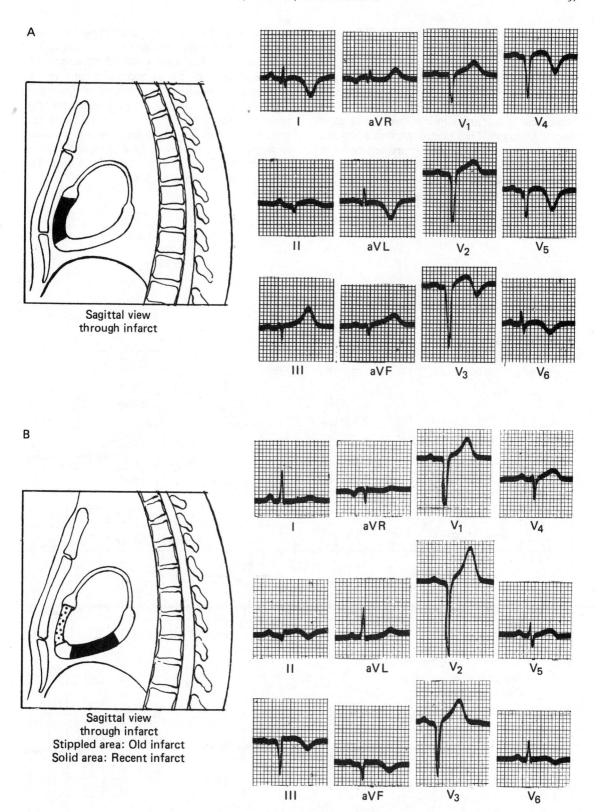

**Figure 10–11.** Multiple myocardial infarctions. *A:* Initial infarction. There are QS complexes in V$_{1-5}$. The T waves are inverted in I, aVL, and V$_{3-6}$. The pattern indicates anterior wall myocardial infarction, and the pattern was stable for several months. *B:* Second infarction. A deep Q wave with inverted T wave is now present in aVF, indicating inferior wall infarction. As a result, the T waves that were previously inverted in the precordial leads have now become upright.

## VENTRICULAR ANEURYSM
### (Akinesis & Dyskinesis)

An aneurysm of the left ventricle, in which a portion of the ventricular wall is fibrotic and thinned and does not contract (or even expands) during ventricular systole, may follow myocardial infarction. "Aneurysm" is a pathologic term, however, and describes the morphologic characteristics of the scarred muscle. The functional counterparts of aneurysmal tissue are **akinesis** (lack of motion), and **dyskinesis** (paradoxical bulging motion during ven-

tricular systole). The most consistent electrocardiographic finding in these major wall motion disorders of the ventricle following myocardial infarction is the persistence of ST segment elevation in the epicardial leads reflecting the area of infarction (Figs 10–12 and 10–13). The ST segments may remain elevated for months to years. Since this pattern is seen in only about half of autopsy-proved or surgically-proved cases, the absence of ST elevation does not indicate absence of significant ventricular wall motion disorders.

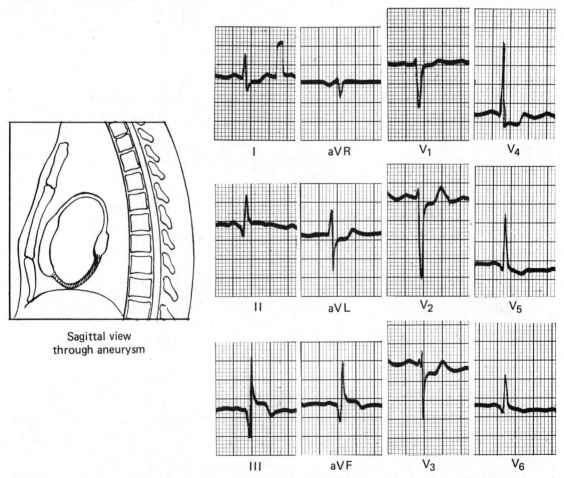

Sagittal view
through aneurysm

I aVR V₁ V₄

II aVL V₂ V₅

III aVF V₃ V₆

**Figure 10–12.** Ventricular aneurysm involving the inferior wall. Deep, wide Q waves with ST segment elevation and T wave inversion are present in II, III, and aVF, indicating inferior wall myocardial infarction. There is ST segment depression in leads I, aVL, and V₁₋₄. Although the ECG might suggest recent inferior wall infarction, this had been a stable pattern over 1 year, and the inferior wall ventricular aneurysm was confirmed by cineangiography and at surgery.

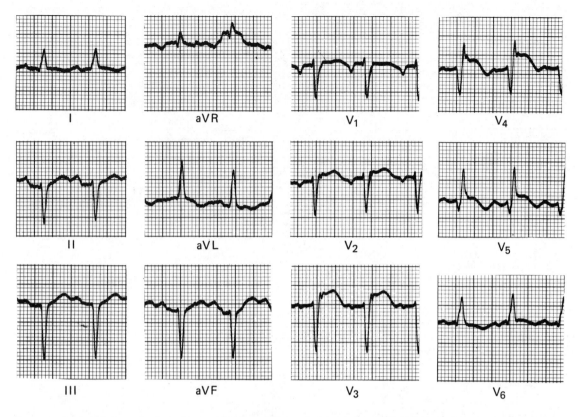

**Figure 10–13.** Anterior ventricular aneurysm. The frontal plane axis is −60 degrees, indicating left anterior fascicular block. There is a diminutive r wave in $V_3$ and wide Q waves in $V_{5-6}$. The ST segments are elevated in $V_{3-5}$. Although this is consistent with acute anterior wall infarction, clinically, the infarction had occurred 1 year before, and serial ECGs had shown no change. A large anterior ventricular aneurysm was documented by left ventricular angiography.

## DIFFERENTIAL DIAGNOSIS OF MYOCARDIAL INFARCTION

### Normal Electrocardiogram

The criterion for an abnormal Q wave is a duration of at least 0.04 s or a Q:R ratio equal to or exceeding 25% (or both). These criteria are not valid for the diagnosis of myocardial infarction if they are present in lead III alone, as up to 35% of normal persons may have these findings. The additional finding of T wave inversion in this lead is also of no diagnostic value (Fig 10–14). Recording lead III during deep inspiration and expiration has been recommended as a means of identifying the inconstancy of Q waves in this lead, but neither its sensitivity nor its specificity for the absence of myocardial infarction is known.

QS complexes may occasionally be seen in $V_2$ in normal individuals (Fig 10–15).

### Left Ventricular Hypertrophy

In hypertrophy of the left ventricle, the left ventricular forces are directed leftward, inferiorly, and posteriorly. Thus, QS complexes may be inscribed in $V_{1-2}$ and are occasionally present through $V_4$. Anterior wall myocardial infarction cannot be read from the ECG with certainty, even though it cannot be excluded as having occurred (Fig 10–16). In addition, the ST segment depression in I, aVL, and $V_{5-6}$ and the ST segment elevation in $V_{1-3}$ associated with left ventricular hypertrophy may further mimic myocardial ischemia or infarction, but they cannot be interpreted as such.

In patients with marked hypertrophy of the interventricular septum, abnormal Q waves can be recorded in many leads, simulating anterior, inferior, lateral, or posterior wall myocardial infarction. Since the normal q wave is due in part to septal depolarization, septal hypertrophy will accentuate this initial force. In addition, the distorted anatomy of the myocardial fibers can contribute to abnormal and delayed impulse conduction through septal tissue. Coronary arteriographic and autopsy data have proved the absence of myocardial infarction in such patients with abnormal q waves.

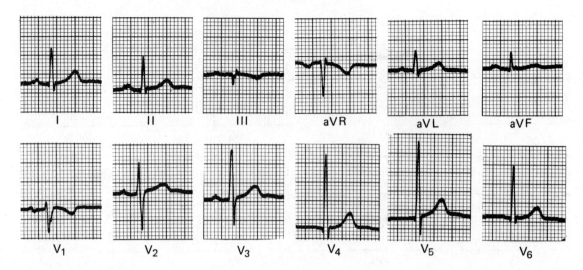

**Figure 10–14.** Normal ECG. There is a Q wave in lead III, and the T wave is inverted in this lead; no other abnormalities (specifically, in leads II and aVF) are present. Such a tracing should not be interpreted as showing inferior wall myocardial infarction.

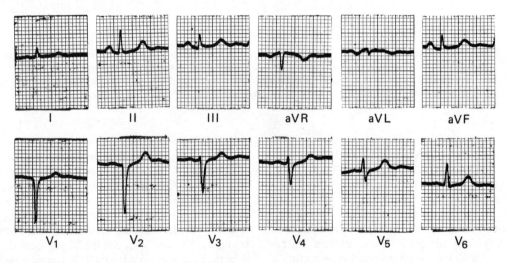

**Figure 10–15.** Normal electrocardiographic pattern with QS complexes in $V_{1-2}$. The R waves progressively increase in height, and the R:S ratio changes appropriately from $V_{3-6}$. There are no ST–T abnormalities. Although old anteroseptal myocardial infarction could have occurred, this sort of tracing is best interpreted as being within normal limits, depending upon the clinical circumstances.

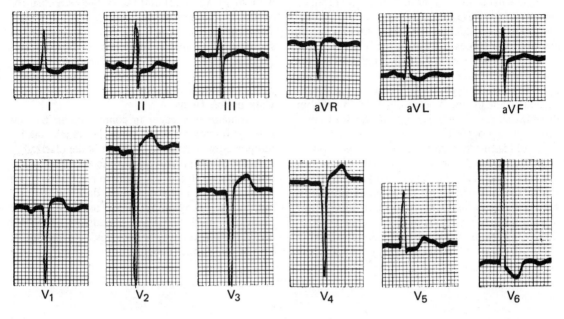

**Figure 10–16.** Left ventricular hypertrophy in a patient with aortic regurgitation. The R wave in aVL is 13 mm, and $SV_1 + RV_6$ is 47 mm. Associated ST elevation is present in leads $V_{1-3}$ and ST depression in I, aVL, and $V_{5-6}$. QS complexes are present in $V_{1-4}$. In the presence of left ventricular hypertrophy, criteria for myocardial infarction cannot be accurately applied.

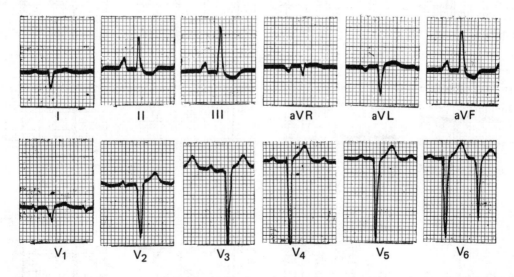

**Figure 10–17.** Right ventricular hypertrophy in a patient with severe chronic obstructive pulmonary disease. QS complexes ae present in leads $V_{1-3}$, representing recordings made over a greatly dilated right ventricle. The progression of R waves over the precordium is poor for the same reason. The P waves are tall and peaked in leads II, III, and aVF, and there is marked rightward deviation of the mean frontal plane QRS axis. This ECG could represent extensive anterolateral wall myocardial infarction (old, because of the upright T waves); the correct diagnosis depends upon clinical correlation.

## Chronic Obstructive Pulmonary Disease With Right Ventricular Hypertrophy

The presence of chronic lung disease, with associated hyperinflation of the lungs, can produce changes in the ECG that mimic myocardial infarction. A marked reduction or even total absence of anterior QRS forces is most commonly observed, resulting in small r waves or QS complexes in precordial leads $V_{1-4}$ (Fig 10–17). If there is additional right ventricular hypertrophy or acute right ventricular overload, the T waves may be inverted in these leads, further mimicking anterior wall myocardial infarction (Fig 10–18).

For reasons that are not quite clear, pulmonary emphysema may distort the mean frontal plane QRS axis, resulting in an abnormally leftward and superior axis (Fig 10–19). This should not be confused with left anterior fascicular conduction delay, since it is not involvement of the intraventricular conduction system that is causing the left axis deviation but alteration of the QRS vector in the frontal plane caused by the lung disease. In addition, abnormal Q waves or QS complexes can be recorded in leads aVF or I, thus mimicking inferior wall or lateral wall myocardial infarction. If the diagnosis of obstructive pulmonary disease is known, any ECG showing these features should not be interpreted as showing myocardial infarction unless there is clinical correlation.

## Left Anterior Fascicular Conduction Delay

If there is a delay in conduction in the left anterior fascicle of the left bundle branch, the inferoposterior surface of the heart is depolarized in advance of the anterosuperior surface. This initial inferoposterior force may result in inscription of a q wave in leads I and aVL, which does not indicate myocardial infarction but occurs as a result of the fascicular conduction delay. In addition, small (but not wide) q waves may be seen in $V_{1-2}$ as a result of loss of the normal depolarization sequence of the

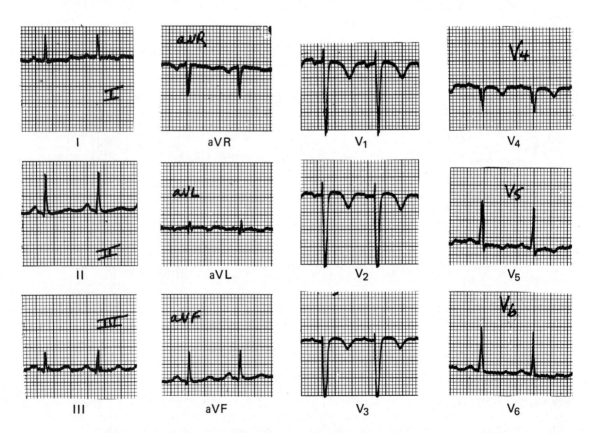

**Figure 10–18.** Acute right ventricular overload due to pulmonary embolism. The ECG shows deep T wave inversion in leads $V_{1-4}$. This electrocardiographic pattern is compatible with acute myocardial ischemia or infarction, but serial tracings failed to show evolution or resolution of the abnormalities, and a lung scan documented a large perfusion defect. Acute pulmonary embolism may be unassociated with rightward axis shift or a change in P wave morphology, with anterior precordial T wave abnormalities the only clue as to its occurrence (as in this case).

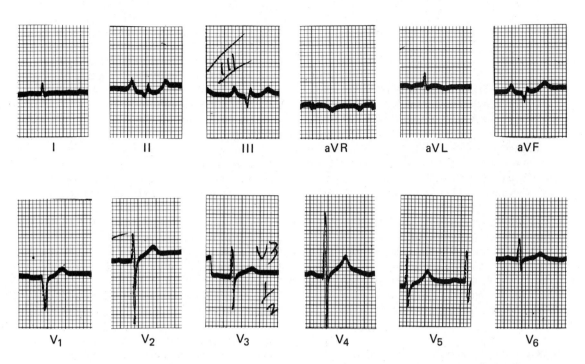

**Figure 10–19.** Right ventricular hypertrophy in a patient with severe chronic obstructive lung disease. The QRS complexes are of low voltage in the frontal plane. Q waves are present in the inferior leads, resulting in superior axis deviation. The P waves are peaked in II, III, and aVF. Inferior wall myocardial infarction was not present at autopsy.

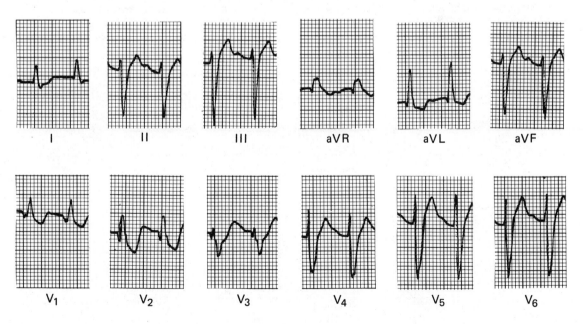

**Figure 10–20.** Left anterior fascicular and right bundle branch block patterns. Anterior wall myocardial infarction is simulated by the small q waves in $V_{1-3}$. These q waves are not due to loss of anterior force resulting from myocardial necrosis but to abnormal septal depolarization caused by conduction delay in the anterosuperior fascicle of the left bundle branch. Left anterior fascicular block is not expected to cause deep, wide Q waves in the precordial leads; when such Q waves occur, they most likely represent myocardial infarction.

anterior portion of the interventricular septum (Fig 10–20).

## MYOCARDIAL INFARCTION WITH DEVELOPMENT OF CONCOMITANT BUNDLE BRANCH BLOCK PATTERNS

In general, a right bundle branch block pattern does not obscure the patterns of myocardial infarction, whereas a left bundle branch block pattern does. The most diagnostic feature of myocardial infarction is the abnormal direction of the initial 0.04-s QRS vector (the Q wave). Since this portion of the QRS complex remains normal in right intraventricular conduction delay, myocardial infarction can be detected when it occurs. However, the initial 0.04-s vector is itself abnormal in left bundle branch block; thus, the infarction pattern is obscured, and the expected abnormal Q wave will not be inscribed.

### Right Bundle Branch Block Pattern & Myocardial Infarction

The concomitant occurrence of right bundle branch block pattern and anterior wall myocardial infarction indicates infarction of the interventricular septum and thus connotes an extensive degree of myocardial necrosis.

As a result of the infarction, the initial r wave of the rSR′ complex in right bundle branch block will disappear in right ventricular epicardial leads, resulting in QR complexes (Fig 10–21). The occurrence of right bundle branch block and inferior wall myocardial infarction suggests that the proximal portion of the right bundle branch, which is supplied by branches of the right coronary artery, is itself ischemic or infarcted. The pattern of inferior wall myocardial infarction is not obscured by the right bundle branch block.

The occurrence of posterior wall myocardial infarction in association with right bundle branch block alters the QRS complexes in the right precordial leads. Conduction delay in the right bundle branch alters the late forces of ventricular depolarization, and posterior wall infarction alters the initial forces of ventricular depolarization. The initial forces of ventricular depolarization are oriented in an abnormally anterior direction. The late forces (the R′) reflecting the right bundle branch conduction delay are also oriented anteriorly. Thus, an abnormally tall, wide R or rR′ wave will be inscribed in the right precordial leads (Fig 10–22). A similar pattern may be seen in patients with right ventricular hypertrophy and right intraventricular conduction delay and also in patients with right bundle branch block alone; thus, confirmatory evidence of myocardial infarction (usually involvement of the inferior wall) must be sought.

### Left Bundle Branch Block Pattern & Myocardial Infarction

The concomitant occurrence of left intraventricular conduction delay and acute myocardial infarction of either the anterior or inferior wall connotes extensive damage to the interventricular septum. Whether the left bundle branch block pattern is new or old, however, the diagnosis of acute myo-

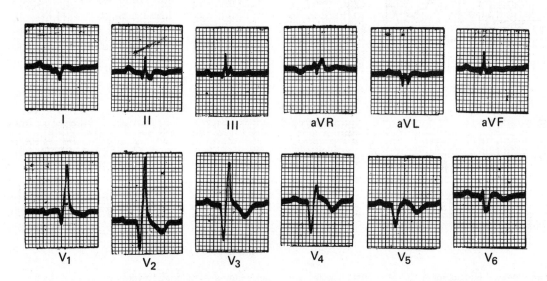

**Figure 10–21.** Anterior wall myocardial infarction associated with right bundle branch block. The QRS duration is 0.14 s, and the VAT in $V_{1-2}$ is 0.1 s. The initial r waves of an uncomplicated right bundle branch block pattern that are normally seen in right precordial leads are not present. Instead, deep wide Q waves indicative of anterior wall myocardial infarction are recorded.

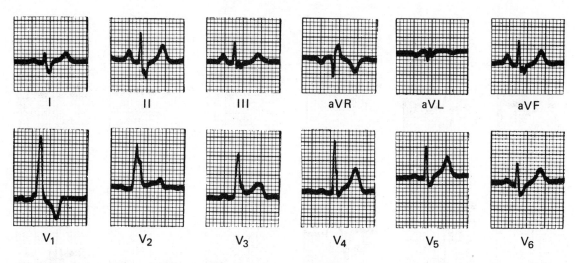

**Figure 10–22.** Posterior wall myocardial infarction and right bundle branch block. The QRS interval is 0.12 s. The wide s waves in leads I, II, III, aVF, and V$_{5-6}$ and the late portion of the R waves in V$_{1-3}$ are indicative of right bundle branch block. The initial tall R deflection in V$_{1-3}$ is consistent with associated posterior wall infarction but not diagnostic of it, since the same pattern can occur in right ventricular hypertrophy or right intraventricular conduction delay.

cardial infarction can be made only infrequently from the ECG. In the presence of left bundle branch block, 2 electrocardiographic findings suggest the diagnosis of acute infarction, which must nevertheless be confirmed by independent means: marked ST segment elevation (Fig 10–23) and the inscription of a new q wave where it is not expected (Fig 10–23). Q waves in association with a left bundle branch block pattern are considered to be due to infarction of the anterior wall, as a result of which a conduction delay distal to the common left bundle occurs (peri-infarction block). An alternative mechanism of the inscription of a q wave in left bundle branch block is extensive infarction of the septum with loss of septal forces; the q wave then represents the forces generated by the free wall of the right ventricle.

The development of the left bundle branch block in a patient with prior infarction obscures the electrocardiographic pattern of the infarction, which can then no longer be read (Fig 10–24).

## TRANSIENT Q WAVES

Although abnormal Q waves are virtually diagnostic of myocardial infarction, they occasionally appear only transiently (Fig 10–25). The conditions in which transient Q waves may be observed include coronary artery spasm and shock states. The

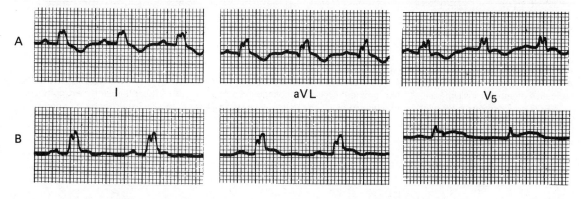

**Figure 10–23.** Myocardial infarction in the presence of left bundle branch block pattern. **A:** Prior to acute infarction. A left bundle branch block pattern is present; note the q wave in lead aVL, which suggests anterior infarction or a component of peri-infarction conduction delay. **B:** Recorded during an episode of severe chest pain. ST segment elevation is present in leads I, aVL, and V$_5$. Independent confirmation of myocardial infarction is required. (In this patient, infarction was confirmed by diagnostic elevations of serum creatine kinase MB fractions.)

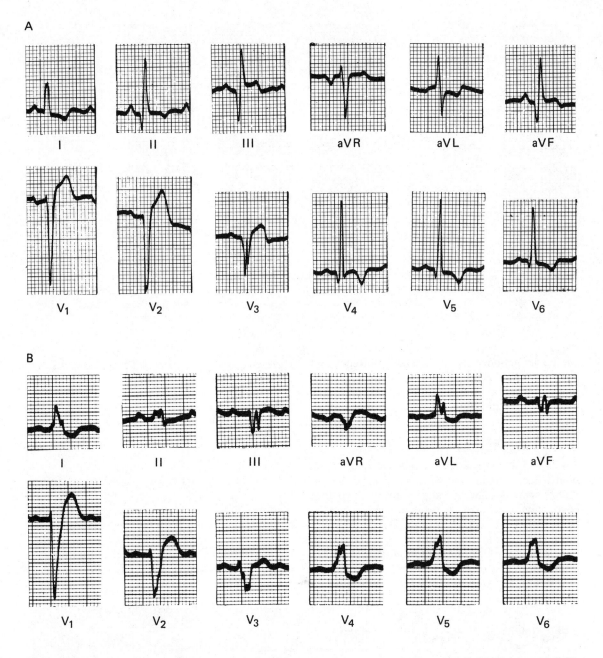

**Figure 10–24.** Infarction associated with left bundle branch block. *A:* The deep, wide Q waves with ST–T changes in II, III, and aVF are indicative of inferior wall infarction. The QS complexes in $V_{2-3}$ and abnormal q waves with T inversion in $V_{4-6}$ are indicative of anterior wall infarction. The prominent precordial voltage is compatible with left ventricular hypertrophy. *B:* This ECG now demonstrates a left bundle branch block and voltage suggesting left ventricular hypertrophy; the previous signs of infarction are no longer seen.

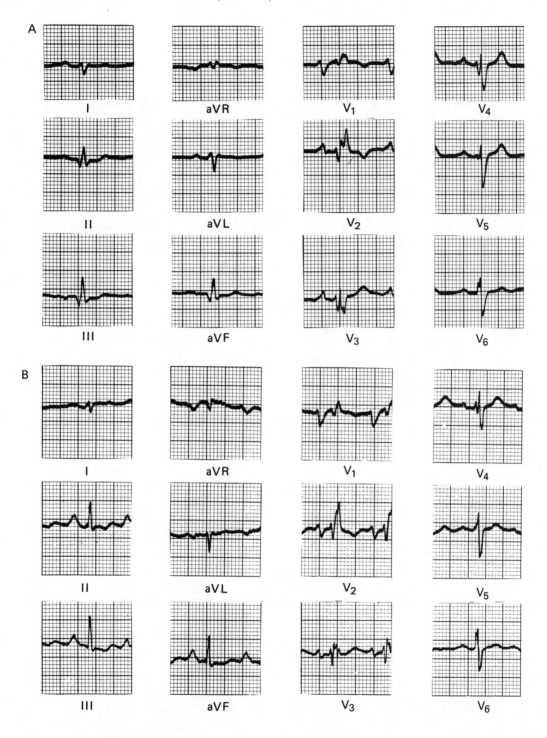

**Figure 10–25.** Transient abnormal Q waves. *A:* The rhythm is sinus. The PR interval = 0.24 s, indicating first-degree AV block. The notched P waves in the frontal plane leads and the diphasic P with a wide negative deflection in $V_1$ are consistent with left atrial abnormality. The QRS interval = 0.15 s, and there is a wide S in I and wide, notched R′ waves in $V_{1-2}$, indicating right bundle branch block pattern. Wide Q waves are seen in II, III, and aVF and are consistent with inferior wall infarction. *B:* Taken 1 day after (A). The QRS interval is reduced to 0.12 s, but the right bundle branch block persists. Q waves are no longer present in II and aVF. Clinical data: The patient had mitral stenosis. At the time of tracing (A), he was in shock as a result of thromboembolism of the abdominal aorta. At the time of tracing (B), his blood pressure and peripheral perfusion had been temporarily improved. It is concluded that the Q waves seen in (A) resulted from severe myocardial ischemia, which subsided at the time of record (B). Autopsy findings: Mitral stenosis with left atrial and right ventricular hypertrophy; extensive thrombosis of abdominal aorta; no myocardial infarction; no pulmonary embolization.

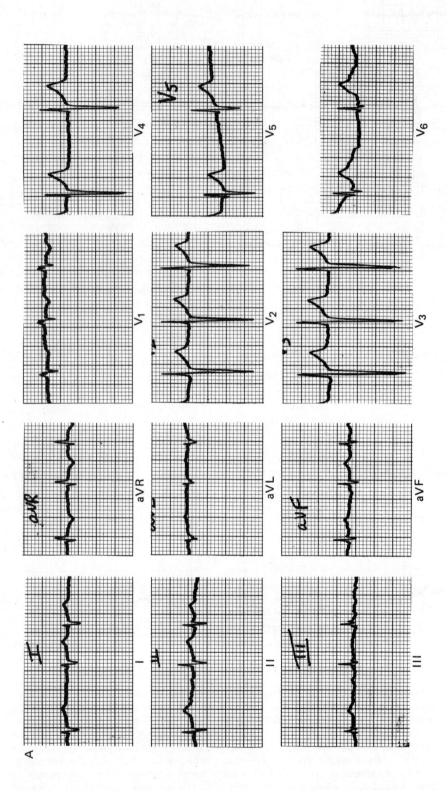

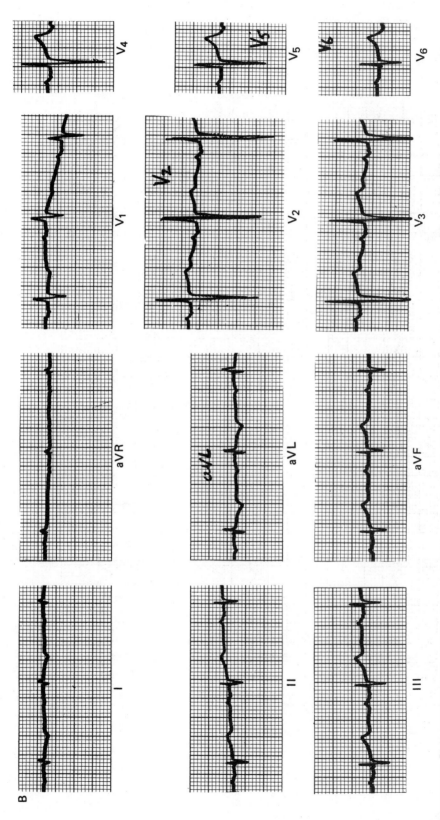

**Figure 10–26.** Right ventricular hypertrophy due to mitral stenosis. **A:** The rhythm is atrial fibrillation. The mean frontal plane QRS axis is +120 degrees. There is a prominent R wave in $V_1$, with an R:S ratio approaching 1.0. **B:** ECG recorded after mitral valve replacement and direct current cardioversion. Sinus rhythm is present. A new Q wave with inverted T wave is present in lead I, suggesting lateral wall myocardial infarction. However, the P wave is also inverted in lead I and aVL, providing a clue to the diagnosis of lead misplacement. Leads II-III and aVR-aVL are reversed as a result of accidental interchange of the RA and LA electrodes.

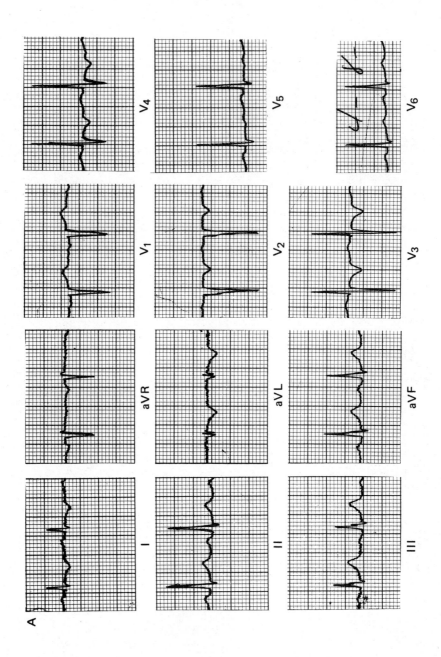

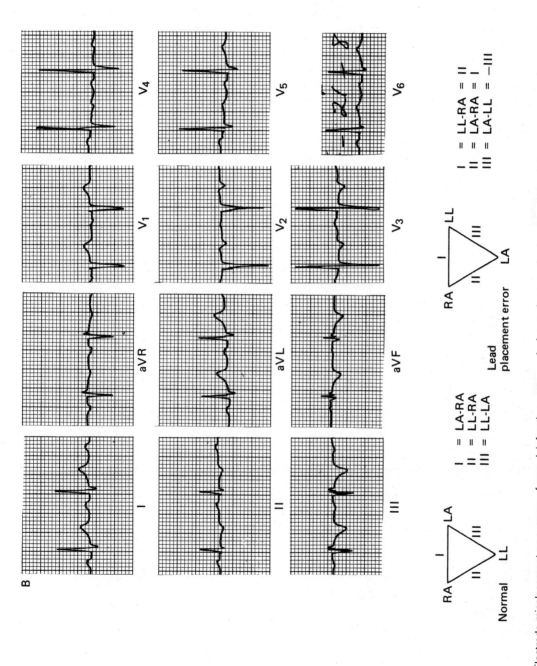

**Figure 10–27.** Electrode misplacement as a cause of pseudoinfarction pattern. *A:* Anterior wall myocardial infarction (QS complex in V₂, qRS complex in V₃, and T wave inversion in V₂₋₄) of uncertain age (clinically known to have occurred 3 years earlier). *B:* As a result of accidental interchange of the LA and LL electrodes, a pseudoinfarction pattern is present in the inferior leads. The diagram illustrates the resultant effect of LA-LL lead reversal.

reason for the appearance and disappearance of the abnormal Q wave is not understood, but it is possible that transient, reversible, severe myocardial ischemia is the unifying underlying cause.

## PSEUDOINFARCTION DUE TO INCORRECT LEAD PLACEMENT

The interchange of RA, LA, and LL electrodes can result in marked changes in the frontal plane leads, mimicking myocardial infarction (Figs 10–26 and 10–27). Lead misplacement will not alter the P–QRS–T configurations in the precordial leads, because the indifferent electrode is the sum of the potentials of RA + LA + LL, irrespective of the individual locations on the extremities.

## PERIPHERAL CONDUCTION DELAYS IN ASSOCIATION WITH MYOCARDIAL INFARCTION (Peri-infarction Block)

Infarction of the myocardium can involve fibers from the anterior and posterior fascicles of the left bundle branch as they radiate over the anterosuperior and inferoposterior surfaces of the ventricle, respectively, as well as the more distal Purkinje fibers. Conduction delay that is limited to the area surrounding the infarction zone is termed **peri-infarction block.** The QRS complexes that show the infarction pattern will therefore appear to be more prolonged than QRS complexes recorded from areas remote from the infarction; notching may be present (Fig 10–28). Peri-infarction block should not be misinterpreted as fascicular block, which involves the fascicles of the left-sided conduction system. Fascicular block will produce axis deviation in the frontal plane and does not itself prolong the QRS duration, whereas in peri-infarction block the frontal plane QRS axis is not altered and the QRS duration appears lengthened over the leads that show q waves.

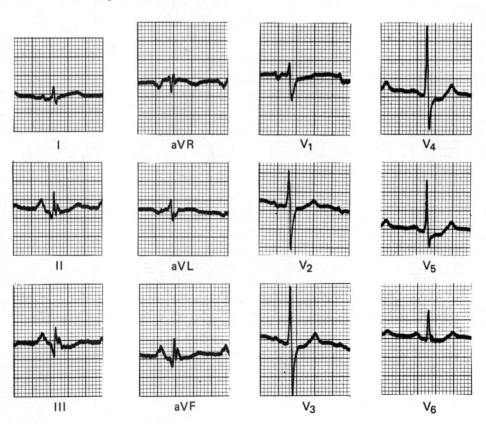

**Figure 10–28.** Peri-infarction block recorded in the inferior leads, occurring as a result of inferior wall myocardial infarction. The QRS duration in the inferior leads is 0.12 s, and the complexes are notched. There are Q waves in II, III, and aVF, and the terminal QRS forces are oriented inferiorly (notched R waves in II, III, and aVF) and slightly rightward (small s wave in I). Although the mean frontal plane QRS axis of +60 degrees suggests the possibility of left posterior fascicular block, the prolongation of the QRS interval makes peri-infarction block a more likely diagnosis.

## TEST TRACINGS

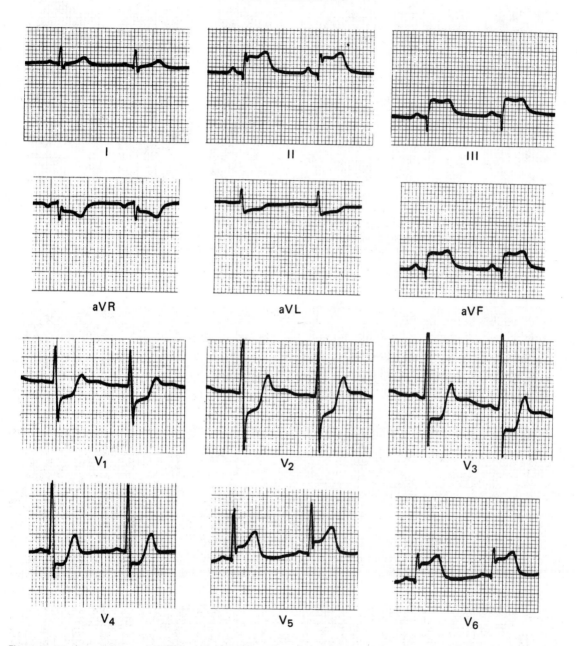

**Figure 10–T1.** Acute inferoposterolateral myocardial infarction. ST elevation is present in leads II, III, aVF, and $V_{5-6}$, and ST depression is present in aVL and $V_{1-4}$. Q waves are present in II, III, and aVF. There is a tall R wave in lead $V_1$, reflecting loss of posterior forces and consequent accentuation of anterior forces in the anterior precordial leads. The ST segment depression in $V_{1-4}$ may reflect reciprocal changes to posterior wall ST elevation or anterior wall ischemia.

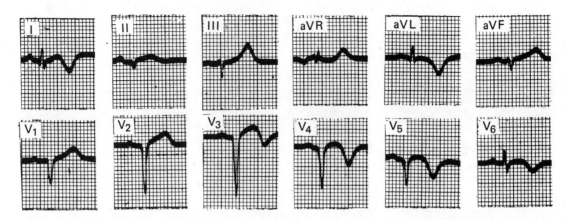

**Figure 10–T2.** Anterior wall myocardial infarction (uncertain age) with left axis deviation, indicating left anterior fascicular block. The rhythm is sinus, the PR interval = 0.16 s, and the QRS duration = 0.06 s. The mean frontal plane QRS axis = −40 degrees. QS complexes are present in $V_{1-5}$, and T wave inversion is present in I, aVL, and $V_{3-6}$. This pattern is most compatible with recent infarction, although similar patterns can persist for years after the event.

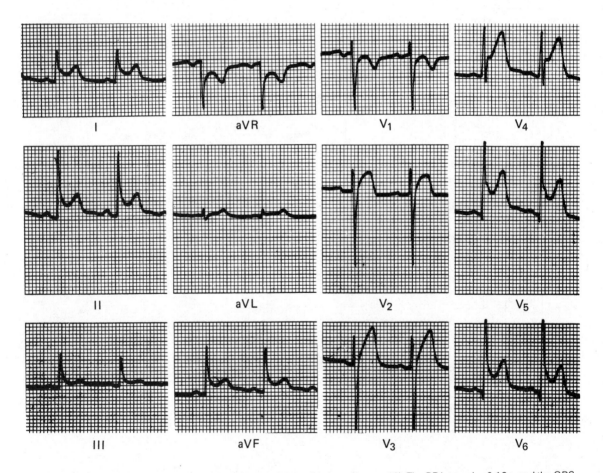

**Figure 10–T3.** Acute pericarditis due to staphylococcus endocarditis (see Chapter 19). The PR interval = 0.16 s, and the QRS duration = 0.08 s. There is concave ST segment elevation in leads I, II, III, aVF, and $V_{2-6}$. The ST segment is isoelectric in aVL and depressed in aVR and $V_1$. This ECG suggests acute transmural myocardial ischemia or infarction, but the widespread nature of the ST–T abnormalities should suggest a diffuse process such as pericarditis. Clinical correlation and serial ECGs would be required to arrive at the correct diagnosis.

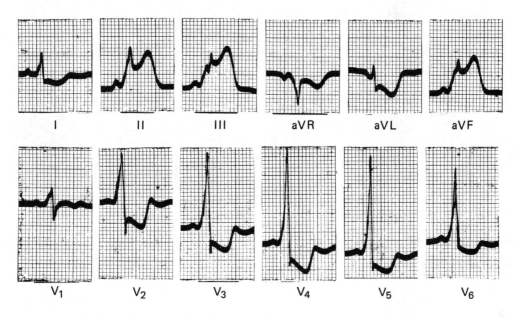

**Figure 10–T4.** Acute inferior wall myocardial infarction and delta waves indicating Wolff-Parkinson-White conduction (see Chapter 16). The rhythm is sinus, the PR interval = 0.10 s, and the QRS duration = 0.12 s. The delta wave slurs the upstroke of the R wave in leads I, II, III, and aVF and all precordial leads. The "R" wave in $V_1$ is not due to posterior wall myocardial infarction but represents the delta wave (pseudoinfarction pattern). In Wolff-Parkinson-White conduction, left ventricular depolarization and repolarization are abnormal, thus precluding the electrocardiographic diagnosis of myocardial infarction; however, in this case the marked ST segment elevation in the inferior leads strongly suggests the diagnosis.

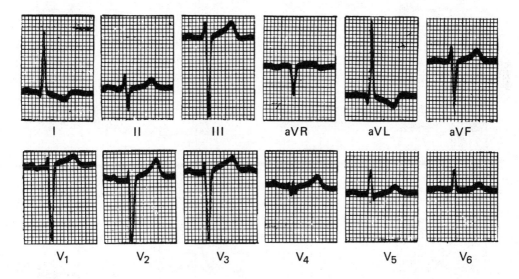

**Figure 10–T5.** Left ventricular hypertrophy. The rhythm is sinus, the PR interval = 0.16 s, and the QRS duration = 0.08 s. The mean frontal plane QRS axis is borderline at −30 degrees. There is downsloping ST depression in leads I and aVL. The R wave voltage in aVL is about 20 mm. Prominent, but not pathologic, q waves are seen in I and aVL. The precordial leads show loss of R wave voltage in lead $V_4$. In left ventricular hypertrophy the left ventricular forces are directed leftward, inferiorly, and posteriorly. Thus, poor progression of R waves and even loss of R waves may be seen in the precordial leads. A prominent q wave in leads I and aVL may be due to depolarization of a hypertrophied interventricular septum or, in part, to associated left axis deviation. Anterior myocardial infarction may thus be mimicked by left ventricular hypertrophy.

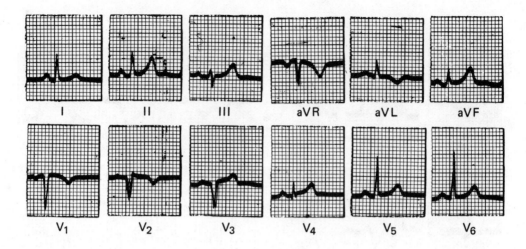

**Figure 10–T6.** Anterior wall myocardial infarction. The rhythm is sinus, the PR interval = 0.14 s, the QRS duration = 0.06 s, and the mean frontal plane QRS axis = +30 degrees. QS complexes are present in $V_{1-3}$ with an abrupt transition to a left ventricular epicardial complex in $V_4$. The T waves are inverted in leads aVL and $V_{1-2}$.

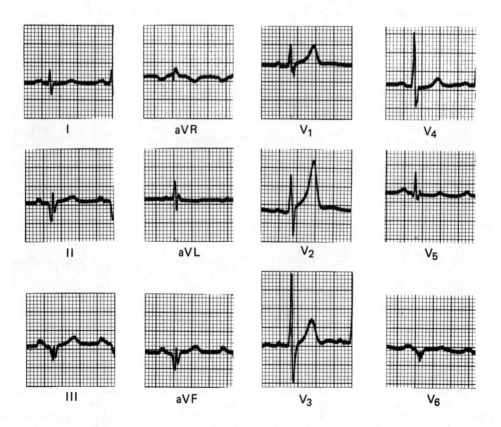

**Figure 10–T7.** Inferoposterior myocardial infarction (old). The rhythm is sinus, the PR interval = 0.16 s, and the QRS duration = 0.10 s. Deep, wide Q waves are seen in II, III, and aVF, and a notched QS complex is seen in $V_6$. A tall R wave is present in $V_1$, with an R:S ratio of 4:1. The T waves are upright in $V_{1-3}$. The tall R wave in $V_1$ reflects loss of posterior forces, with accentuation of anterior forces as recorded from the anterior precordial leads. The age of the infarction is judged to be old from the upright T waves in the inferior leads.

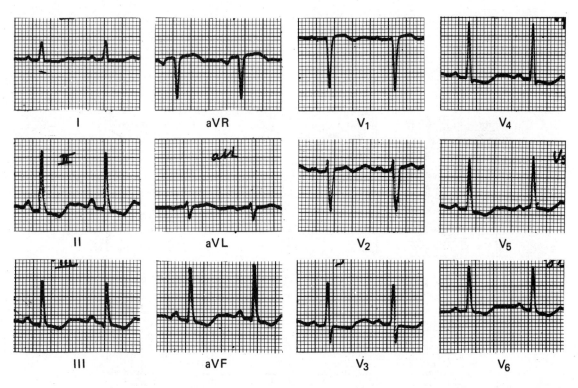

**Figure 10–T8.** Nondiagnostic ST –T wave abnormalities in a patient taking phenothiazine medication (see Chapter 17). The rhythm is sinus, the PR interval = 0.18 s, the QRS duration = 0.08 s, and the mean frontal plane QRS axis is +70 degrees. ST segment depression is present in leads II, III, aVF, and $V_{3-6}$. A prominent U wave is present, which prolongs the QTU interval. The QRS complexes are normal. Although these ST –T wave abnormalities might suggest myocardial ischemia or infarction, they must be considered to be nonspecific if there is no confirmatory evidence of these processes.

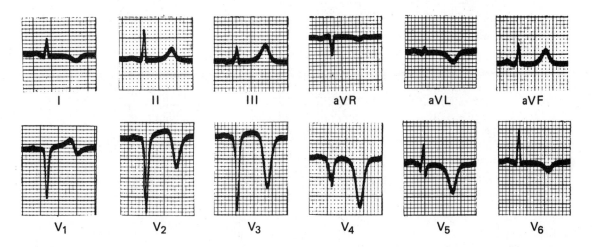

**Figure 10–T9.** Anterior wall myocardial infarction of indeterminate age. The rhythm is sinus, the PR interval = 0.14 s, the QRS duration = 0.08 s, and the mean frontal plane QRS axis = +60 degrees. There are QS complexes in $V_{1-4}$, and a qR complex in $V_5$. Deep, symmetric T wave inversion with mild ST segment elevation is present in leads I, aVL, and $V_{2-6}$. This pattern is occasionally seen within hours of acute myocardial infarction but more commonly occurs within weeks after the event and may remain for the rest of the patient's life.

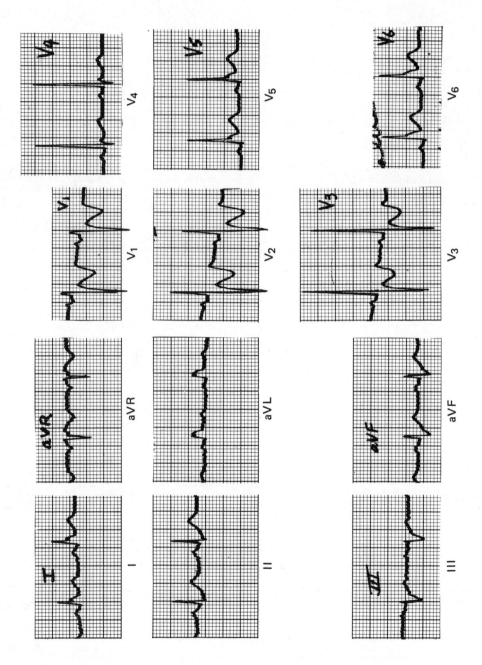

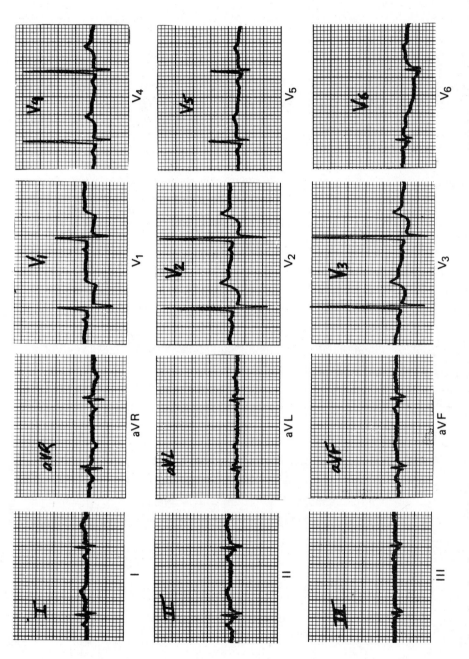

**Figure 10–T10.** Acute inferoposterolateral wall myocardial infarction. *A:* Marked ST segment depression is present in $V_{1-3}$ and ST elevation in $V_{5-6}$. In addition, there is notching of the terminal portion of the R wave in leads I and $V_{5-6}$, suggesting a distal left ventricular conduction delay (peri-infarction block). *B:* Tracing recorded 24 hours later. Q waves have now appeared in leads II, III, aVF, and $V_6$, and the ST segment abnormalities are resolving. Tall R waves have now appeared in $V_{1-2}$.

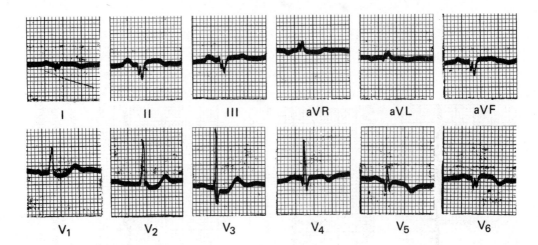

**Figure 10–T11.** Inferoposterolateral wall myocardial infarction. The rhythm is sinus, the PR interval is 0.14 s, and the QRS duration is 0.08 s. The mean frontal plane QRS axis is −100 degrees, reflecting the loss of inferior forces (rather than conduction delay in the left anterior fascicle of the left bundle branch). Notched QS complexes with inverted T waves are seen in leads I, II, aVF, and $V_6$. The T wave is inverted in $V_{4-5}$. Tall R waves are present in $V_{1-2}$, reflecting the loss of posterior forces. Right ventricular hypertrophy as a cause of the prominent anterior forces is unlikely under these circumstances, in which myocardial infarction may be diagnosed from other aspects of the ECG, but it should still be excluded on clinical grounds.

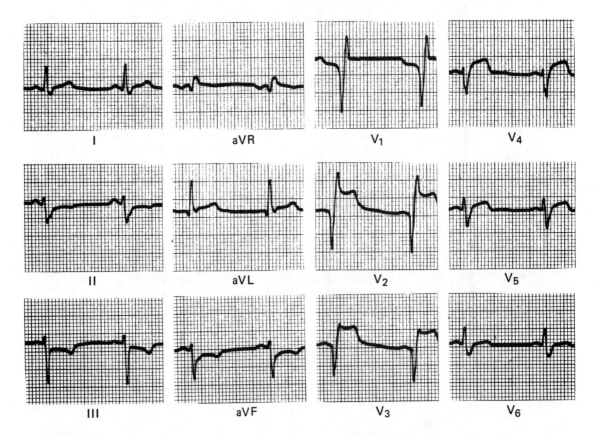

**Figure 10–T12.** Left anterior fascicular conduction delay, right bundle branch block pattern, and anterior wall myocardial infarction. Deep, wide Q waves are present in $V_{1-3}$. Such Q waves are too deep and too broad to be the result of the anterior fascicular block. In addition, ST segment elevation in $V_{1-4}$ and ST segment depression in II, III, and aVF confirm the acute myocardial infarction.

# Normal Cardiac Rhythm & the Supraventricular Arrhythmias | 11

## PHYSIOLOGY OF CARDIAC RHYTHM

Activation of heart muscle results from spontaneous impulse formation occurring in a pacemaker cell and conduction of this impulse from cell to cell. Disturbances of cardiac rhythm are related to the basic processes of automaticity, conduction, and triggering.

### Automaticity

Cells that are capable of pacing the heart have the property of automaticity, the basis for which is the spontaneous depolarization of the cell during phase 4 (see Chapter 2). Normally, the sinus node serves as the pacemaker for the heart, since its phase 4 depolarization is the most rapid and thus its automatic rate is the fastest. However, should the firing rate of the sinus node slow below that of other, subsidiary pacemaker cells, these *escape* pace-

makers will take over the pacing function of the heart. Pacing tissue is present within the specialized conduction system of the heart—portions of atrial tissue, areas in the AV junction, the common bundle of His, the bundle branches, and the peripheral Purkinje system.

The rate at which pacemaker cells discharge depends on the following: (1) the membrane potential present at the end of repolarization, (2) the slope (rate) of phase 4 diastolic depolarization, and (3) the threshold potential at which the cell is able to be depolarized. Lowering the membrane potential away from the threshold potential, slowing the slope of phase 4, or raising the threshold potential toward zero all slow the firing rate of the pacemaker cell; whereas raising the membrane potential toward the threshold potential, increasing the slope of phase 4, or lowering the threshold potential so that it is closer to the membrane potential all increase the

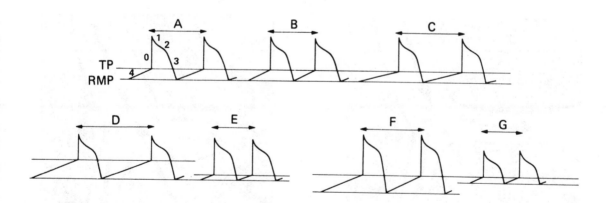

**Figure 11–1.** Schematic drawing of action potentials and the determinants of intrinsic firing rate. Phase 4 represents diastolic depolarization; RMP, resting membrane potential; and TP, threshold potential. *A:* Impulse formation is determined by the slope of phase 4 and by the levels of RMP and TP. *B:* An increase in the slope of phase 4 results in an increase in firing rate (enhanced automaticity). *C:* A decrease in the slope of phase 4 results in a decrease in firing rate (decreased automaticity). *D:* Raising the threshold potential toward 0 mV, resulting in a longer time required until the cell achieves threshold and is activated, with a consequent decrease in automaticity. *E:* Lowering the threshold potential toward resting membrane potential, resulting in less time required for the cell to reach threshold and depolarize (enhanced automaticity). *F:* Lowering of resting membrane potential away from threshold potential, resulting in a longer time required for threshold to be reached (decreased automaticity). *G:* Raising of resting membrane potential closer to threshold potential, requiring a shorter time necessary to attain threshold (enhanced automaticity).

firing rate (Fig 11–1). Variables that affect the automaticity of pacemaker cells are listed in Table 11–1.

## Conductivity

The ability of cardiac tissue to conduct an impulse (conductivity) is dependent upon phase 0 (the rate of change of voltage) and the amplitude of the action potential. Slowing the rate of phase 0 or decreasing the amplitude of the action potential (or both) decreases the speed of conduction of an impulse through the tissue (conduction delay) and favors the development of failure of impulse transmission (conduction block). A progressive decrease

**Table 11–1.** Variables that affect automaticity of pacemaker cells.*

| Increased Firing Rate | Decreased Firing Rate |
|---|---|
| Sympathetic nervous system activity | Parasympathetic nervous system activity |
| Hypoxia | Hypothermia |
| Hypercapnia | Hyperkalemia |
| Cardiac dilatation | |
| Ischemia/necrosis | |
| Hypokalemia | |

*These variables affect both automaticity and conduction properties of different portions of the specialized conduction system to varying degrees; thus, the net effect on pacemaker rate will depend upon their interaction.

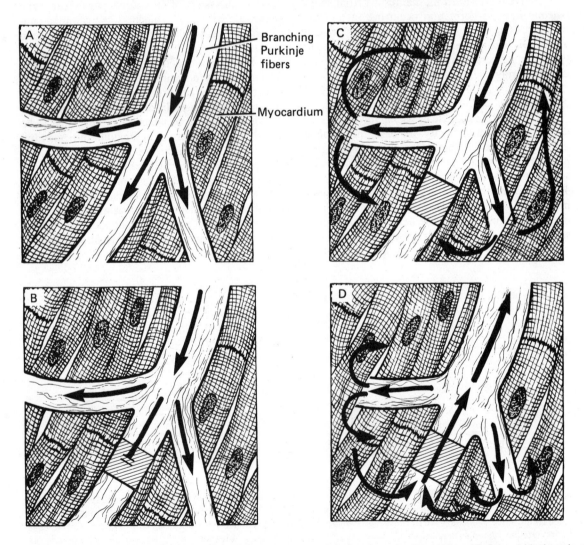

**Figure 11–2.** Schema of a reciprocating arrhythmia caused by decremental conduction, with unidirectional block and reentry. *A:* Normal propagation of an impulse through branching Purkinje fibers, with activation of the neighboring myocardium. *B:* A zone of decremental conduction (hatched area) causes unidirectional block of the impulse. *C:* Propagation of the impulse through normally conducting fibers activates the myocardium. *D:* The impulse that has spread through the myocardium penetrates the zone in which depressed antegrade conduction was present and is propagated in a retrograde direction, thus reactivating the Purkinje fibers and producing a second (reentry or reciprocating) response. Maintenance of this circuit leads to reciprocating tachyarrhythmias.

in the rate of rise of phase 0 and the action potential amplitude leads to **decremental conduction,** in which impulses fail to be conducted further.

If decremental conduction occurs in only one direction (unidirectional block), an impulse that has failed to be conducted in that direction may be capable of being propagated in the opposite direction, thus initiating a reciprocating (or reentry) arrhythmia (Fig 11–2).

**Concealed conduction** occurs when an impulse penetrates a portion of the conduction system (most commonly the AV junction) but is not propagated further; its presence is inferred from its effects on subsequent electrocardiographic events.

### Triggering

Triggered activity refers to cell depolarizations that are initiated by a drive stimulus that produces an action potential that displays an ''afterdepolarization'' wave (Fig 11–3). An afterdepolarization wave is actually a voltage oscillation. It may occur early or late relative to the action potential. If early, the afterdepolarization has occurred before complete repolarization of the cell; if late, the afterdepolarization has occurred after complete repolarization of the cell. If the afterdepolarization waves reach threshold, the cells can depolarize spontaneously for a brief period of time. Digitalis toxic rhythms, as well as some catecholamine-stimulated arrhythmias, are thought to be due to triggering.

## THE SINUS RHYTHMS

The P waves in an ECG represent atrial depolarization. Actual pacing activity occurring within the sinus node precedes atrial depolarization and is therefore not seen in the ECG. That P waves are sinus-stimulated is therefore inferred from their morphology.

**Sinus rhythm** is the normal cardiac rhythm, and its rate is usually 60–100/min. **Sinus tachycardia** is present when the sinus rate exceeds 100/min, although with exercise the sinus rate can approach 200/min. **Sinus bradycardia** is present when the sinus rate is less than 60/min. Neither sinus tachycardia nor sinus bradycardia per se indicates organic heart disease.

**Sinus arrhythmia** is present when the sinus rate varies with respiration, with slower rates being present during expiration and more rapid rates during inspiration. It is not an abnormal rhythm and is more common in young subjects. Fig 11–4 illustrates the sinus rhythms.

The sinus P wave has a mean frontal plane axis of between +15 and +75 degrees and is thus upright in I, II, and aVF, inverted in aVR, and variable in III and aVL. In the horizontal plane the sinus P wave may be inverted in $V_1$ but is upright in $V_{3-6}$. Some variability in sinus P wave contour in III and aVF may be present with respiration.

**Sinoatrial block** exists when not all impulses generated by the sinus pacemaking cells leave the SA node to reach the atrial conducting tissue and depolarize the atria. In the absence of atrial depolarization, a P wave will not be inscribed on the ECG. SA block may take the form of progressive delay in transmission of the impulse through the sinus node to the atrium, resulting in a nonconducted sinus impulse (SA Wenckebach, or type I, exit block [see Chapter 12]) or abrupt failure of transmission of the impulse to the atrium (type II SA exit block [see Chapter 12]). Abrupt failure of conduction can take the form of 2:1, 3:1, etc, SA block. High-degree SA block will manifest itself on the surface ECG as pauses in sinus rhythm, which cannot always be differentiated from either sinus arrest due to failure of impulse generation or from atrial standstill due to inability of the atrial muscle to be depolarized. Only

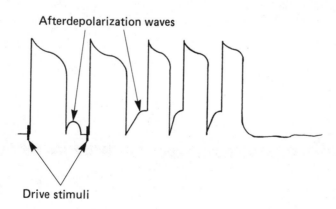

Afterdepolarization waves

Drive stimuli

**Figure 11–3.** Schema of a triggered rhythm. The first driven action potential is followed by a small afterdepolarization wave. The second drive stimulus is followed by an action potential with a sufficiently large afterdepolarization wave to reach threshold, initiating (triggering) a self-terminating burst of tachyarrhythmia.

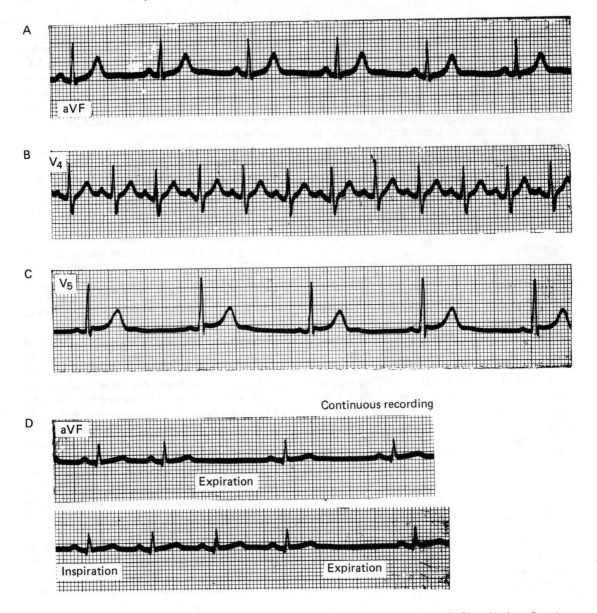

**Figure 11–4.** *A:* Normal sinus rhythm, rate = 63/min. *B:* Sinus tachycardia, rate = 125/min. *C:* Sinus bradycardia, rate = 50/min. *D:* Sinus arrhythmia with increase in rate during inspiration and decrease during expiration. The P wave contours are identical.

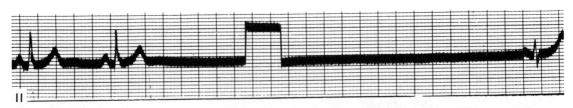

**Figure 11–5.** Pause in sinus rhythm of 4.6 s. The pause is terminated by a sinus P wave conducted to the ventricles aberrantly. The pause is not a multiple of the basic sinus rate and could therefore be due to failure of impulse generation within the sinus node. Atrial standstill, in which the atrial muscle is incapable of being depolarized despite being stimulated, is also a possibility if underlying sinus arrhythmia is assumed.

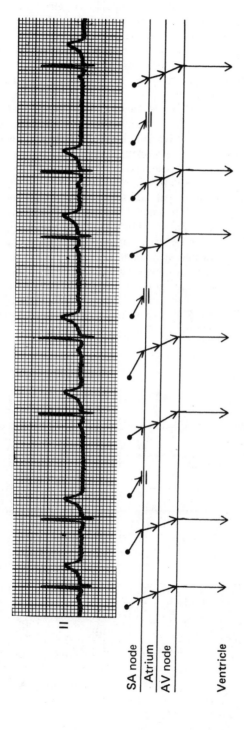

**Figure 11–6.** Sinus node exit block (3:2 type I [Wenckebach] block). Repetitively, 2 sinus-conducted impulses are followed by a pause. All P waves are of the same configuration, the PR intervals are constant, and no nonconducted atrial premature beats are evident. In type I SA exit block, the sinus node fires regularly (but cannot be seen in the ECG). The impulses encounter progressive delay in exiting the sinus node until one is not conducted to the atrium. In this instance, every third sinus impulse fails to be conducted to the atrium.

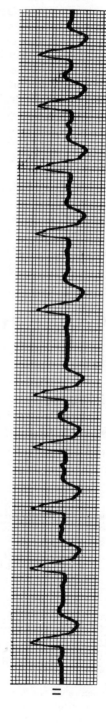

**Figure 11–7.** Type I (Wenckebach) SA exit block. Cycles of 5 sinus-conducted impulses are followed by a pause. The PR intervals are constant. The PP interval between the first 2 beats of the cycle is longest because the greatest increment of conduction delay occurs between the first 2 beats of the Wenckebach period (see Chapter 12). Left bundle branch block is also present.

if the pauses between sinus P waves are multiples of a basic sinus rate is the diagnosis of type II SA block tenable. Figs 11–5 through 11–7 illustrate these points.

**Sinoventricular conduction** is the term used to describe sinus impulses that are conducted through the atrial conduction system and into the AV node but which fail to depolarize atrial tissue. This type of conduction is seen principally in hyperkalemia, which causes atrial muscle standstill even though intra-atrial conduction is preserved (Fig 11–8). Since the atria are not depolarized, the surface ECG shows QRS complexes without preceding P waves. Measures that increase sinus rate might result in an increase in QRS rate, but the diagnosis can be made with certainty only if P waves that occur at the same rate as the prior QRS rhythm appear when the hyperkalemia is being treated (Fig 11–8).

## ABNORMAL ATRIAL RHYTHMS

### Atrial Premature Beats

An atrial premature complex (P′ wave) results from an impulse arising in an ectopic focus in the atria. As the impulse is premature, atrial excitation is early relative to the sinus rate. An atrial premature impulse will usually initiate ventricular activation and produce a QRS complex, which may be normal or aberrant (see Chapter 8), depending upon whether the bundle branches are refractory at the time of arrival of the impulse. An atrial premature impulse may be so early as to meet refractoriness in the AV node, in which case no QRS complex results and the impulse is said to be nonconducted (Figs 11–9 and 11–10). Nonconducted atrial premature impulses are the most common cause of pauses in cardiac rhythm.

The P′ wave contour will depend upon the focus of origin of the impulse and on the intra-atrial spread of activation. Generally, atrial premature beats that arise near the sinus node have a normal mean frontal plane axis (upright in I, II, and aVF; negative in aVR) (Fig 11–11); those arising in the lower portion of the atrium have a superior axis (negative in II and aVF and upright in aVR), as the atria are depolarized in retrograde fashion (Fig 11–12), and those arising in the mid portion of the atria have an intermediate axis.

The P′R interval depends upon the distance of the focus of origin of the ectopic impulse to the AV node as well as on the RP′ interval that precedes it. Thus, the P′R interval may be longer or shorter than the sinus PR interval.

Continuous recording

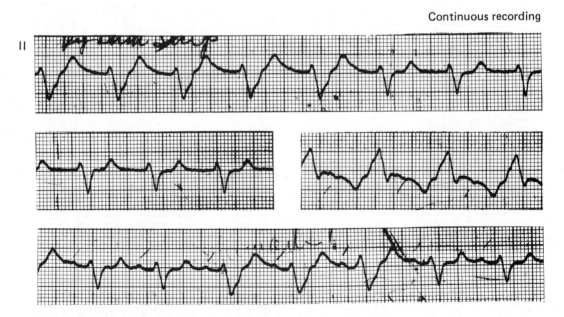

**Figure 11–8.** Probable sinoventricular conduction in a patient with hyperkalemia (serum K⁺ = 6.7 meq/L). In the top strip, the rhythm appears to be junctional (or ventricular) in origin, since no P waves precede the broad QRS complexes. Respiratory variation in the QRS duration is present. In the middle strip, P waves emerge and precede the QRS complexes at regular PR intervals of about 0.19 s. The P wave rate is the same as the QRS rate in the top strip, suggesting that sinus impulses stimulated the QRS complexes by traversing the interatrial conduction pathways to enter the AV node–His-Purkinje system. Since atrial muscle is more sensitive to the effects of hyperkalemia than conduction system fibers, atrial muscle depolarization does not occur despite intact interatrial impulse conduction, and thus P waves are not inscribed in the ECG.

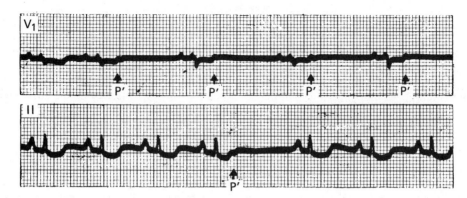

**Figure 11–9.** Nonconducted atrial premature impulses. In the $V_1$ rhythm strip, the first 2 beats are sinus, and the PP interval is 0.68 s. A P' occurs in the T wave of the second QRST complex, with a PP' interval of 0.36 s. Since the P' wave occurs so early, it encounters refractoriness in the AV node–His-Purkinje system because of normal conduction of the previous sinus impulse; the P' impulse is therefore not conducted (blocked). In the lead II rhythm strip, a P' occurs in the T wave of the fourth QRS complex. It is not conducted because of its prematurity.

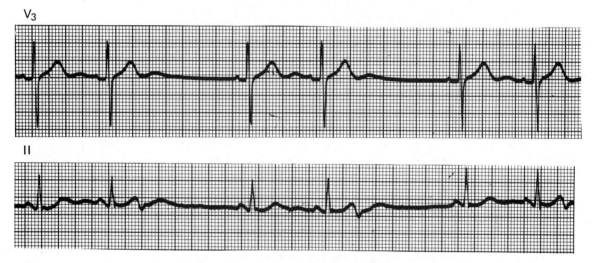

**Figure 11–10.** Nonconducted atrial premature complexes. The recorded leads $V_3$ and II illustrate the point that not all ECG leads show events equally well. Groups of 2 sinus beats are followed by a pause. Whereas in lead $V_3$ the pause appears to result from sinus arrest, in lead II premature P' waves are clearly seen in the T waves of the second of the pair of sinus beats. This grouping, in which 2 sinus beats are followed by an atrial premature beat, is called "atrial trigeminy."

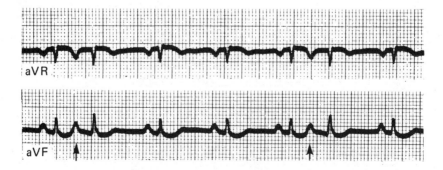

**Figure 11–11.** The rhythm is predominantly sinus at a rate of 75/min (the PP interval is 0.8 s). The P' waves occur 0.64 s after preceding P waves and thus are premature (arrows). The P'R interval is longer than the sinus PR interval, reflecting delayed AV nodal conduction due to conduction of the preceding atrial impulse. Since the P' waves are inverted in aVR and upright in aVF, the focus of origin is high in the atrium.

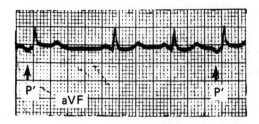

**Figure 11–12.** Sinus rhythm at a rate of 80/min is present. The premature P' waves are inverted in aVF, suggesting a focus of origin low in the atrium with retrograde atrial depolarization. Since the premature P' wave falls late in diastole, it does not encounter delay in the AV node, and the P'R interval is therefore normal.

Nonconducted P' impulses are followed by pauses that are described as "fully compensatory" or "less than fully compensatory." If the premature impulse fails to penetrate the sinus node, the sinus firing rate continues undisturbed, and the interval from the sinus beat preceding the atrial premature beat to the next sinus beat will equal two PP intervals. If the premature impulse penetrates the sinus node, it discharges the sinus pacemaker cells prematurely and resets their cycle. Since the sinus node is discharged early and reset, the interval between the sinus beat preceding the atrial premature beat and the next sinus beat will be less than two PP intervals. Pauses that are less than fully compensatory or fully compensatory depend only upon whether or not the

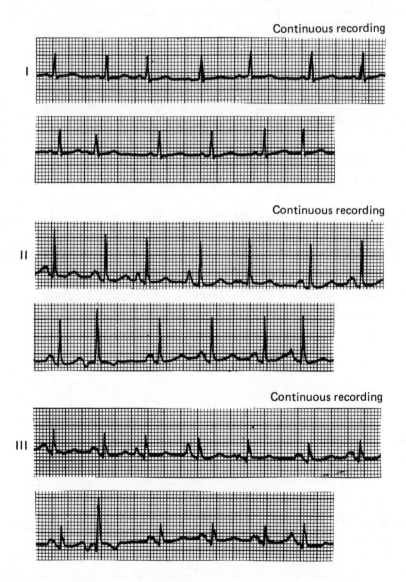

**Figure 11–13.** Wandering pacemaker. Each QRS complex is preceded by a P wave, but the P wave contours vary, as do the PR intervals. Changing P wave contours reflect the different foci of origin of the P waves. Identification of a given P wave as originating in the sinus node is not always possible.

sinus node has been penetrated by an ectopic impulse and not by the site of origin of that impulse.

## Wandering Atrial Pacemaker

In this arrhythmia, some atrial impulses originate in the sinus node and others in various portions of the atria and AV junction. Thus, multiple P wave contours and variability in atrial rate and PR intervals are seen (Fig 11–13).

## Multifocal Atrial Tachycardia

Multifocal atrial tachycardia, as its name implies, is an atrial arrhythmia characterized by varying P wave contours reflecting different foci of origin and by variable PR intervals (Figs 11–14 and 11–15). It is similar to wandering atrial pacemaker, but the rate is faster, exceeding 100/min and often reaching 130/min. Occasionally, P waves are not conducted to the ventricles because of their prematurity. Often, intraventricular conduction is aberrant. Multifocal atrial tachycardia is most commonly seen in patients with chronic obstructive pulmonary disease or severe congestive heart failure. It is important to recognize this rhythm, as it is easily confused with atrial fibrillation yet does not respond to digitalis therapy, which may mistakenly be given in toxic doses in an attempt to slow the ventricular rate.

## Ectopic (Automatic) Atrial Tachycardia

Ectopic atrial tachycardia is an automatic rhythm arising in an atrial focus. Its rate is usually 150–200 and may be slightly irregular. The usual AV conduction ratio is 1:1, but Wenckebach type I AV block or type II AV block can occur, depending upon the tachycardia rate and integrity of AV conduction (Fig 11–16) (see Chapter 12). The P′R interval is often prolonged because of the rapid atrial rate and also possibly because of abnormal atrial and AV nodal depolarization pathways.

The ectopic P′ waves are generally directed inferiorly and leftward, resulting in a normal P′

axis. However, they are characteristically peaked and of brief duration, thus distinguishing them from sinus P waves. An ectopic atrial rhythm arising near the sinus node, however, may not be easily distinguishable from sinus tachycardia. Carotid sinus massage may be of value in differentiating between the two: Sinus tachycardia is expected to slow slightly, whereas the rate of an atrial tachycardia will not change even though AV block with slowing of ventricular rate is produced. (In contrast, AV nodal reentry tachycardia may be abolished by carotid sinus massage, as the AV block produced by the maneuver disallows reentry of the tachycardia impulse within AV nodal tissue [see below].)

## Atrial Flutter

Atrial flutter is a regular atrial rhythm resulting from intra-atrial reentry or "circus movement" of impulses. The rate is usually 220–350 but may be as low as 175 or as high as 430. Slow atrial flutter rates occur in patients with large or hypertrophied atria and in those receiving quinidine. The most commonly observed atrial rate is 300/min. The AV conduction ratio of the flutter impulses is usually 2:1 or 4:1 in patients receiving no treatment; thus, the ventricular rate is usually regular at 150/min or 75/min (Fig 11–17). However, because of varying AV conduction ratios as well as type I (Wenckebach) block at the AV node, the ventricular rate in atrial flutter may be irregular.

The atrial waves in atrial flutter (F waves) are characteristically "saw-toothed" in appearance, reflecting atrial depolarization and repolarization ($T_a$) waves. This characteristic morphology is most easily seen in leads II, III, and aVF and may not be apparent at all in $V_1$ or may mimic ectopic atrial tachycardia in this lead (Fig 11–17). In other leads, the F waves may resemble the wavy baseline of atrial fibrillation (Fig 11–17). Carotid sinus pressure will result in AV block of some of the flutter impulses, allowing the atrial waves to be more

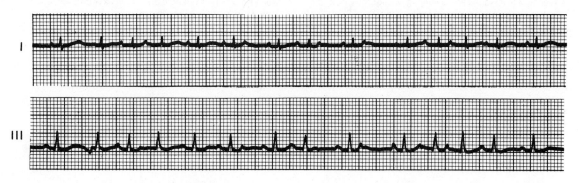

**Figure 11–14.** Multifocal atrial tachycardia. The ventricular rhythm is irregular at about 140/min. Each QRS is preceded by a P wave, but P wave contours and PR intervals vary. Some P waves are not conducted to the ventricles.

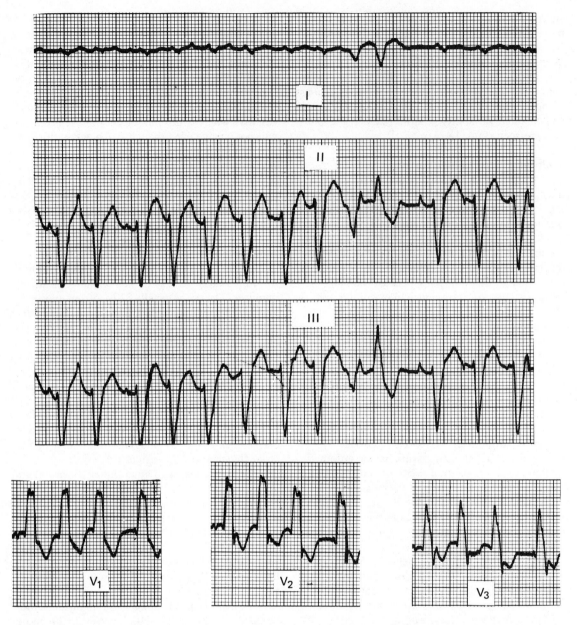

**Figure 11–15.** Multifocal atrial tachycardia. The ventricular rate is irregular at about 130/min. Each QRS is preceded by a P wave, but the P waves are of varying configurations, and the PR intervals vary. Right bundle branch block is present, and the superior axis deviation is compatible with left anterior fascicular block. Further intraventricular aberration is seen in the ninth and tenth QRS complexes in the simultaneously recorded leads I, II, and III.

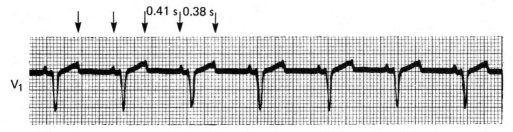

**Figure 11–16.** Atrial tachycardia with 2:1 AV conduction. The ventricular rhythm is regular at 75/min. The atrial rate varies: the PP intervals enclosing a QRS complex are 0.38 s and the PP intervals not enclosing a QRS complex are 0.41 s (arrows). This phenomenon, in which the PP intervals vary depending upon the presence or absence of QRS complexes, is termed **ventriculophasic arrhythmia** and is thought to result from reflex mechanisms induced by the ventricular contraction resulting from the QRS complex. Whereas in this $V_1$ lead the rhythm suggests atrial tachycardia with block, confirmation of the atrial mechanism requires analysis of the atrial waves in II, III, and aVF to exclude the saw-toothed pattern of atrial flutter, which can occasionally occur at this slow rate.

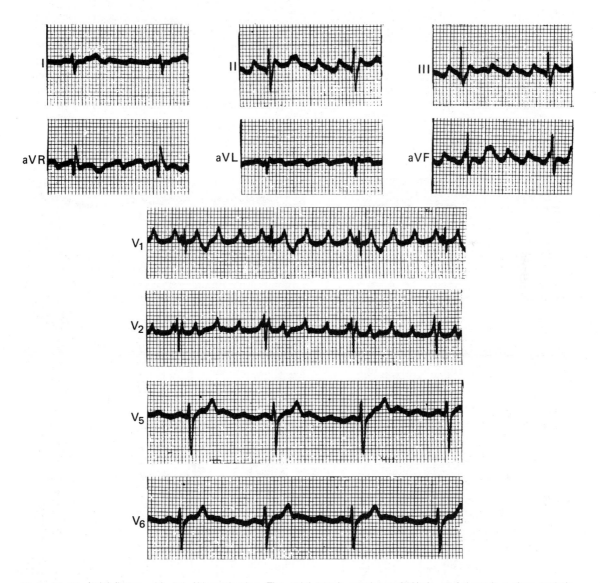

**Figure 11–17.** Atrial flutter with 4:1 AV conduction. The atrial rate is regular at 240/min, and there is a characteristic "saw-toothed" appearance to the flutter waves that is best seen in leads II, III, and aVF. In contrast, the atrial waves do not have this appearance in the precordial leads, where atrial tachycardia ($V_1$) or atrial fibrillation ($V_6$) might be mimicked.

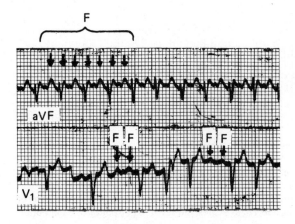

**Figure 11–18.** Atrial flutter with 2:1 AV conduction and a ventricular rate of 215/min. If the flutter wave at the end of the QRS complex is not appreciated, this rhythm might suggest ectopic atrial tachycardia. However, the identification of 2 atrial waves for each QRS complex and the sawtoothed appearance of the F waves in aVF indicate atrial flutter. With carotid sinus massage (lower strip), clear flutter waves are discerned as further AV block of some of the impulses is produced.

clearly seen and the correct diagnosis of the atrial rhythm to be made (Fig 11–18).

## Atrial Fibrillation

Atrial fibrillation is a very rapid irregular rhythm. Most of the fibrillatory impulses (f waves) fail to be propagated through the AV node to the bundle of His (decremental conduction) to stimulate the ventricles; thus, the ventricular response is irregular and occurs at rates as low as 50/min and as high as 200/min in the unmedicated patient. The ventricular response to atrial fibrillation depends upon the integrity of AV nodal conduction and autonomic nervous system input, with sympathetic stimulation increasing the ventricular rate and parasympathetic stimulation decreasing it.

Atrial fibrillatory waves may be "fine," resulting in a wavy baseline in the surface ECG (Fig 11–19), or "coarse," resulting in defined atrial waves that, although they may resemble atrial flutter waves, are too rapid (Fig 11–20). The latter rhythm has been termed "flutter-fibrillation," "coarse atrial fibrillation," and "impure flutter,"

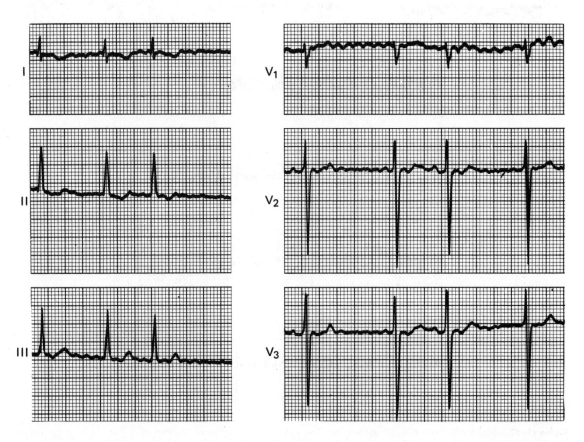

**Figure 11–19.** Atrial fibrillation. Atrial activity is manifested by rapid, small, irregular atrial (f) waves. The ventricular rhythm is irregular.

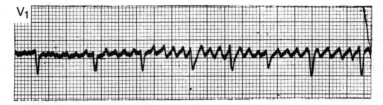

**Figure 11–20.** Atrial flutter-fibrillation. In the first portion of the strip, fine atrial fibrillatory waves are seen. In the latter portion of the strip, the atrial waves have a more organized configuration and appear to occur at regular intervals at a rate of 500/min. This rate is too rapid to be atrial flutter, although another term to describe it is "impure flutter." A hallmark of atrial fibrillation is the variation in contour as well as rate of the fibrillatory impulses.

Continuous recording

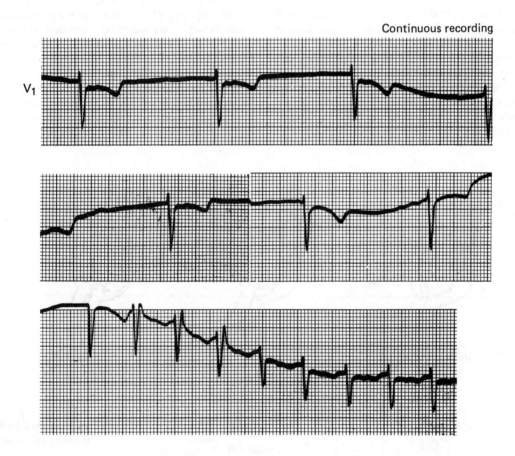

**Figure 11–21.** Bradycardia-tachycardia syndrome. In the top 2 strips, a regular narrow-QRS rhythm is present at a rate of 38/min. The narrow complexes suggest a junctional origin; each complex is followed by a P wave within its T wave, suggesting that retrograde atrial activation is occurring. (However, confirmation of retrograde atrial depolarization must be sought in superior-inferior leads such as II or aVF.) In the bottom strip, a supraventricular tachycardia at a rate of 125/min occurs abruptly; this could be sinus tachycardia or ectopic atrial tachycardia.

but it behaves like atrial fibrillation rather than flutter in its response to treatment. The f waves of atrial fibrillation are usually most prominent in $V_1$, and the saw-toothed configuration of atrial flutter waves is not seen in II, III, and aVF.

### Bradycardia-Tachycardia Syndrome

Bradycardia-tachycardia syndrome is characterized by periods of bradycardia and episodes of supraventricular tachycardia. The bradycardia may be due to sinus arrest or SA exit block, reflecting sinus node dysfunction ("sick sinus syndrome") with subsequent junctional or ventricular escape rhythms. The tachycardias may be ectopic atrial, atrial flutter, atrial fibrillation, or reentry AV nodal tachycardia, singly or in combination (Fig 11–21). The pauses in rhythm are often associated with symptoms of cerebral insufficiency, and cardiac pacing is required. The tachycardias may be associated with palpitations and usually require suppression with antiarrhythmic agents.

Bradycardia-tachycardia syndrome represents a diffuse disease involving the conduction system of the heart but is not necessarily associated with structural heart disease.

## PAROXYSMAL SUPRAVENTRICULAR TACHYCARDIA

Paroxysmal supraventricular tachycardia is characterized by a regular tachycardia, usually occurring at rates of 150–250/min. Unlike ectopic atrial tachycardia, which results from enhanced automaticity of an atrial focus, or triggered atrial arrhythmias, the underlying mechanism of paroxysmal supraventricular tachycardia is more complex (Fig 11–22). In paroxysmal supraventricular tachycardia, a premature impulse fails to propagate down a pathway (unidirectional block) because of a long refractory period in that pathway. The impulse therefore proceeds down a second pathway but is conducted with delay because of slow conduction velocity in this pathway. Because the impulse conducts slowly in the antegrade direction, it has the opportunity to turn around and be conducted retrograde in the first pathway, which has now recovered from its refractory state (Fig 11–22). Maintenance of this "reentry" phenomenon constitutes a reentry, or reciprocating, tachycardia. The tachycardia rate will depend upon the conduction velocity and refractory times of the involved pathways.

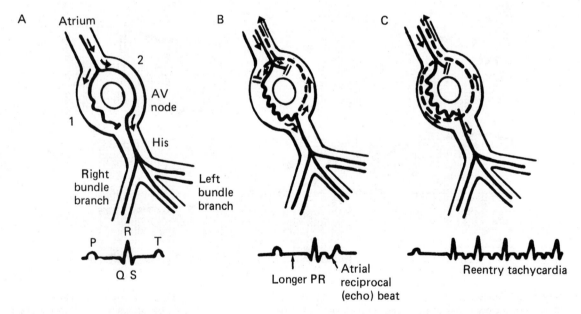

**Figure 11–22.** Schema of a reentry (reciprocating) tachycardia involving 2 pathways in the AV node but which could represent other areas of conduction tissue within the heart. Pathway 1 is capable of conducting an impulse but with delay. Pathway 2 can conduct the impulse without delay but has a long refractory period. *A:* Sinus rhythm, in which the impulse is transmitted down the fast pathway to the ventricles. *B:* A premature impulse fails to be conducted in pathway 2 because of its long refractory period; it is conducted slowly to the ventricles in the slow pathway. The delay in conduction in pathway 1 is manifested by the prolonged PR interval associated with the premature impulse. *C:* Initiation of reentry tachycardia. The premature impulse, which was originally blocked in the fast pathway (pathway 2) and is conducted with delay in the slow pathway (pathway 1), is able to turn around and conduct in retrograde fashion in the fast pathway, which is now no longer refractory. When the impulse reaches a certain level in the reentry pathway, it turns around again and is now conducted in antegrade fashion. Continuation of these events constitutes a reentry (reciprocating) tachycardia.

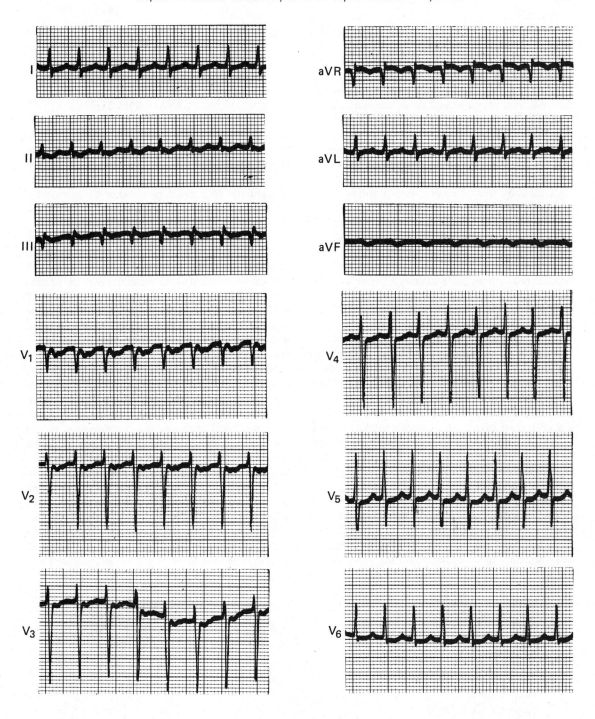

**Figure 11–23.** Paroxysmal supraventricular tachycardia. A regular, narrow complex tachycardia at a rate of 190/min is present. P waves immediately follow the QRS complexes (best seen in V₁ and V₂). Verification of this tachycardia as paroxysmal supraventricular tachycardia would depend upon identifying inverted P waves in the inferior leads.

Paroxysmal supraventricular tachycardias often involve pathways within the AV node itself (AV nodal reentry tachycardia) but may also involve extra-AV nodal bypass tracts (see Chapter 16). In the latter instance, antegrade conduction to the ventricles may proceed down the normal AV node-His-Purkinje system and retrograde conduction via the bypass tract, or antegrade down the bypass tract and retrograde via the normal conduction system. The QRS complex morphology will be determined by the pathway of ventricular depolarization. Most reciprocating tachycardias occur within the AV node.

In AV nodal reentry tachycardia, the surface ECG shows a regular, usually narrow QRS tachycardia (Fig 11–23). The P waves, if they are seen, are inverted in II, III, and aVF, since the atria are depolarized in retrograde manner. The relation of the P waves to the QRS complexes (preceding, superimposed on, or following) depends upon the relative conduction times from the reentry sites (levels) to the atria and ventricles, respectively.

Anything that blocks conduction of impulses within the AV node (such as carotid sinus massage, edrophonium, digoxin, beta-blocking drugs, and some calcium channel-blocking agents) either terminates the paroxysmal supraventricular tachycardia or has no effect, in distinct contrast to such effects in ectopic atrial tachycardia, atrial flutter, and atrial fibrillation, in which the atrial rate and rhythm remain essentially unchanged, although AV block is produced.

Reentry tachycardias are not confined to the AV node or extra-AV nodal bypass tracts but may involve the sinus node (sinus node reentry tachycardia), bundle of His and bundle branches (bundle branch reentry tachycardia), and Purkinje-myocar-

dial tissue (some forms of ventricular tachycardia). Atrial flutter is another form of reentry tachyarrhythmia in which both atria participate.

## JUNCTIONAL RHYTHMS

### Junctional Impulses

The AV node is divided into the atrionodal (A-N) region, the "N" region, and the nodal-His (N-H) region. As the "N" region of the AV node is thought not to contain pacemaker cells, rhythms originating in this area are currently termed "AV junctional" rather than "nodal" rhythms.

Impulses arising in the A-N and N-H regions are conducted to the atria in retrograde fashion, producing inverted P waves in II, III, and aVF. They are conducted to the ventricles over the normal His-Purkinje pathways. The relation between the P waves and QRS complexes will depend upon the relative conduction times from the junctional focus to the atria and ventricles, respectively; thus, the P waves can precede, be superimposed upon, or follow the QRS complexes (Fig 11–24). If the P waves precede the QRS complexes, differentiation from an ectopic atrial rhythm originating in the inferior portions of the atria may not be possible.

Junctional impulses can be premature or can occur as a result of slowing of the sinus rate, in which case they are termed **escape beats.** A junctional premature beat, which results from enhanced automaticity of the AV junction, can initiate an **accelerated junctional rhythm,** which usurps the sinus rate, resulting in AV dissociation (Fig 11–25). A junctional escape beat can initiate a junctional **escape rhythm,** with rates of 35/min to 60/min (Fig 11–26). A junctional impulse can also

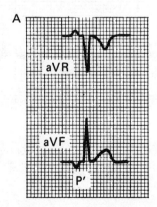 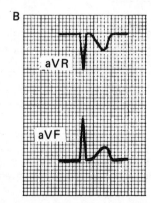 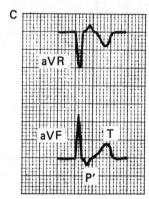

**Figure 11–24.** Electrocardiographic patterns of impulses arising in various sites within the AV junction. *A:* High AV junctional focus (A-N). Note upright P' in aVR and inverted P' in aVF preceding the QRS complex. The impulse is activating the atria before the ventricles. *B:* AV junctional focus. P' buried in QRS complex. The impulse is arising in either the A-N or N-H zones and activating the atria and ventricles simultaneously. *C:* Low AV junctional focus (N-H). Note upright P' in aVR and inverted P' in aVF following the QRS complex. The impulse is activating the ventricles before the atria.

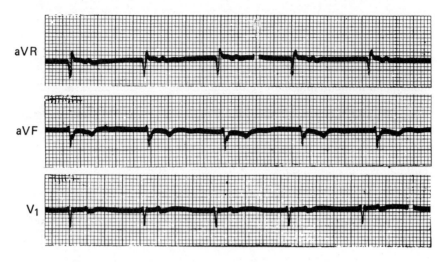

**Figure 11–25.** AV junctional rhythm. A regular QRS rhythm is present at a rate of 70/min. No atrial activity precedes the QRS complexes. P waves are seen in the T waves following each QRS complex. The P waves are upright in aVR and inverted in aVF, indicating retrograde atrial depolarization.

cause a **reciprocal (echo) beat**: If the junctional impulse is conducted slowly in the AV node in retrograde fashion to the atria, it can turn around within the AV node to initiate ventricular activation a second time (Fig 11–26).

### Junctional Tachycardia

Junctional tachycardia is usually due to enhanced automaticity of the AV junction and may be seen as a manifestation of digitalis toxicity or in patients with severe congestive heart failure or those who have had cardiac surgery. Whereas an accelerated junctional rhythm has a rate of 60–120/min, junctional tachycardia has a rate of 120–200/min. Junctional tachycardia may be virtually impossible to differentiate from paroxysmal reentry supraventricular tachycardia on the ECG; however, the clinical circumstances as well as the response to vagal maneuvers (termination of paroxysmal supraventricular tachycardia but no effect on junctional tachycardia) are important distinguishing points.

aVF

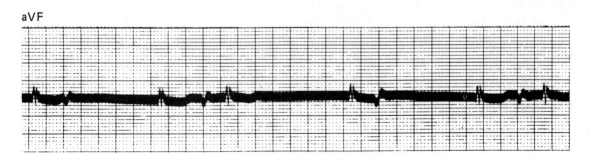

**Figure 11–26.** AV junctional rhythm with retrograde atrial activation and reciprocal ("echo") beats. Each QRS complex is followed by an inverted P wave in its T wave, indicating retrograde atrial activation. The RP' interval is long, reflecting delayed retrograde conduction. The second and fourth retrograde P waves occur at even longer RP' intervals, allowing time for the impulse to turn around within the AV node and be conducted in antegrade fashion to the ventricles ("echo" phenomenon). If these events are sustained, a reciprocating tachycardia could develop.

## TEST TRACINGS

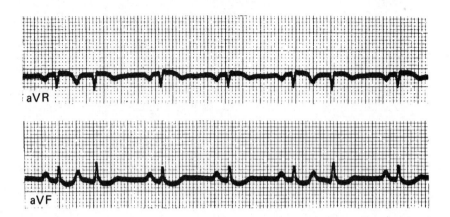

**Figure 11–T1.** Regular sinus rhythm at a rate of 75/min, with atrial premature beats. The P′ waves are inverted in aVR and upright in aVF, occur in constant relationship to the preceding sinus beat **(fixed coupling)**, and deform the T wave of the preceding sinus beat.

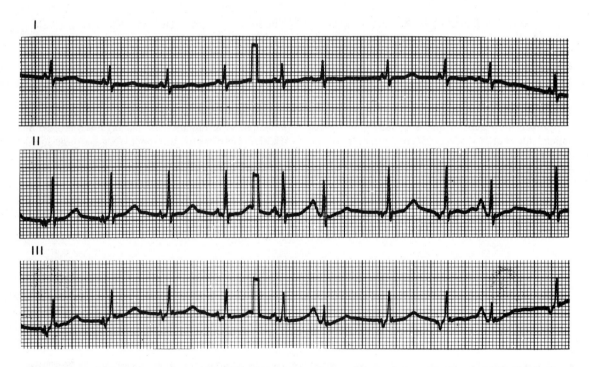

**Figure 11–T2.** Wandering atrial pacemaker. The atrial rhythm is irregular, and the P waves have differing contours. The PR intervals are also variable.

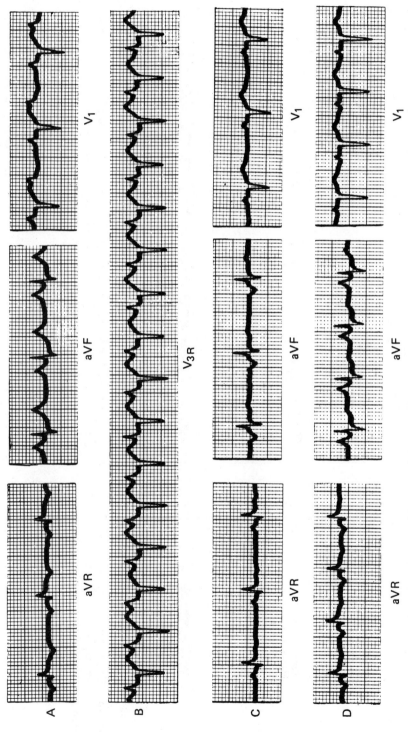

**Figure 11–T3.** This series of tracings was recorded from a patient receiving digitalis. *A:* The atrial rate is 142/min, and the P waves are inverted in aVR and upright in aVF. 2:1 AV conduction is present, which could represent sinus tachycardia with 2:1 AV block or automatic atrial tachycardia with AV block. The latter would be diagnostic of digitalis toxicity. *B:* $V_{3R}$ recorded minutes afterward, shows 1:1 AV conduction with first-degree AV block for this rate. The configuration of the P waves in this lead does not help to distinguish the focus of origin of the atrial rhythm. Digitalis was discontinued. *C:* One day later, the rate is 75/min and 1:1 AV conduction is now present. The P waves are upright in aVR and inverted in aVF, indicating that the atria are being depolarized in a retrograde manner. The rhythm is therefore originating in either the lower portion of the atrium or in the AV junction, with the P' wave preceding the QRS complex because of more rapid retrograde conduction to the atrium than antegrade conduction to the ventricles. *D:* Two days later, sinus rhythm is present at 100/min. The P waves are normally inverted in aVR and upright in aVF. The series represents digitalis toxicity.

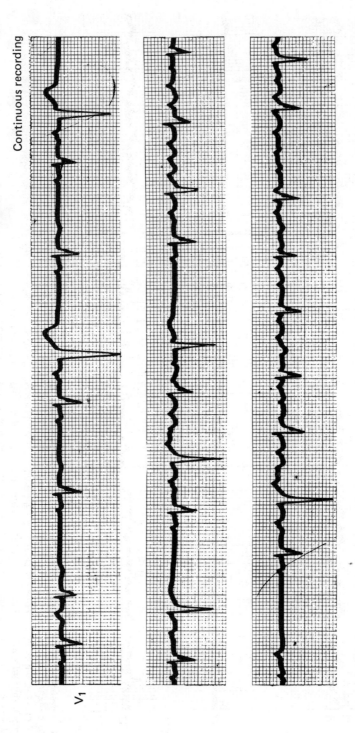

**Figure 11–T4.**  Sinus rhythm with atrial premature complexes is present in the top strip. The atrial premature impulses are conducted to the ventricles aberrantly. In the second strip, atrial premature beats initiate bursts of atrial flutter-fibrillation, 2 of which terminate spontaneously. The initiation of atrial flutter-fibrillation results from an atrial premature impulse falling in the vulnerable period of atrial tissue, similar to the initiation of ventricular tachycardia-fibrillation by a premature ventricular impulse.

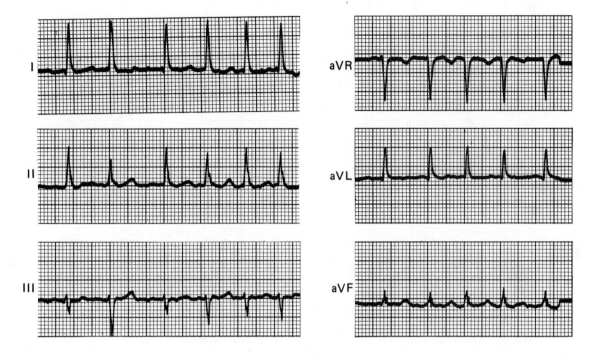

**Figure 11–T5.** Atrial fibrillation. The ventricular rhythm is irregularly irregular. No discrete atrial activity is discernible, but the wavy baseline indicates that the atrial rhythm is fibrillation. Note that the fibrillatory waves are not equally well seen in all ECG leads; when this is the case, the irregularity of the ventricular rhythm is the only clue to the correct diagnosis.

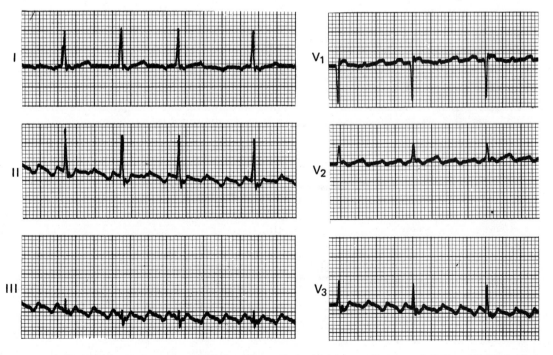

**Figure 11–T6.** The atrial rhythm is regular at 300/min, and saw-toothed atrial waves (best seen in II, III, and aVF) indicate that the rhythm is flutter. Note that the characteristic saw-toothed pattern of atrial flutter is not seen in leads I and V₁. The FR intervals are constant, and the AV conduction ratio varies between 3:1 and 4:1.

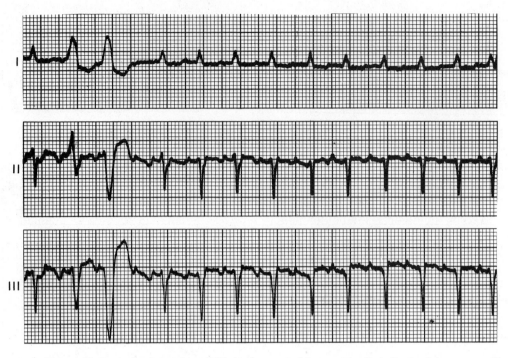

**Figure 11–T7.** The ventricular rhythm is regular at 150/min. For most of the record a single P wave is seen preceding each QRS. The second and third QRS complexes are multiform premature ventricular complexes. The ensuing postextrasystolic pause allows identification of the true atrial rhythm at 300/min. Therefore, the rhythm is atrial flutter with 2:1 AV conduction. Had the premature ventricular beats not allowed correct identification of the atrial rate, the rhythm could have been misdiagnosed as sinus tachycardia or automatic atrial tachycardia. As a general rule, when the ventricular rate is regular at 150/min, atrial flutter with 2:1 AV conduction is present until proved otherwise.

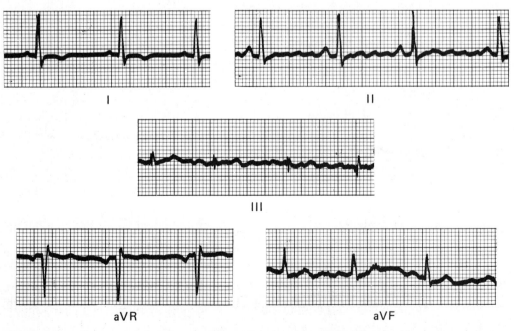

**Figure 11–T8.** Lead III and, to a lesser degree, leads II and aVF show an undulating baseline, suggesting atrial fibrillation. However, leads I and aVR indicate regular sinus rhythm. This ECG was recorded on a patient whose left leg was in a cast. Skeletal muscle contractions of the left leg (which are common to leads II, III, and aVF) explain the artifact in these leads.

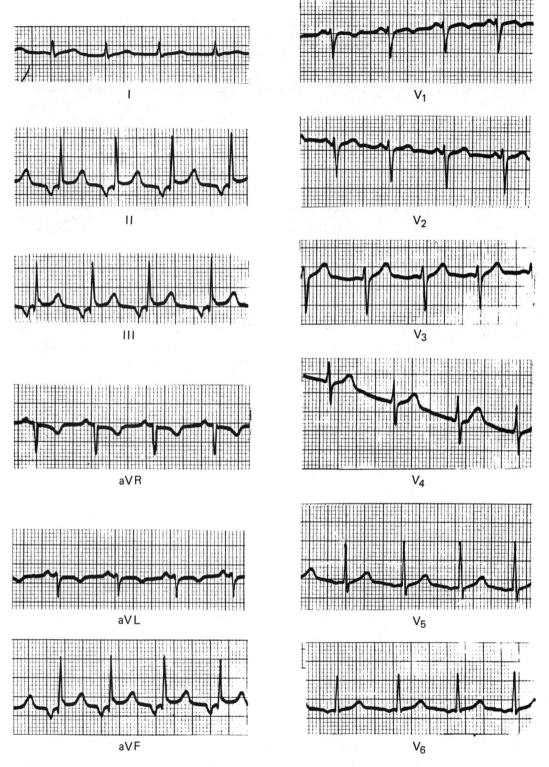

**Figure 11–T9.** Regular rhythm in which each QRS complex is preceded by a P wave at the normal PR interval. The P waves are inverted in II, III, aVF, and V₆, suggesting that the atria are being activated in a retrograde manner. The rhythm could be AV junctional or left atrial in origin; in the latter instance, the P waves would be expected to be inverted in lead I as well.

aVL

aVF

V<sub>1</sub>

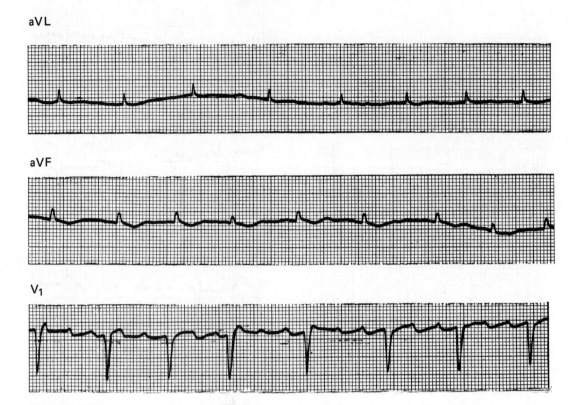

**Figure 11–T10.** Atrial flutter mimicking atrial fibrillation. Atrial activity is not clearly discerned in leads aVL and aVF, and the ventricular rate is not regular. However, V$_1$ shows a regular atrial rhythm at 210/min, with varying AV conduction being responsible for the irregularity of the ventricular rhythm. Irregular ventricular rate without discernible atrial activity suggests atrial fibrillation, but this rhythm is flutter. The relatively slow atrial rate was due to quinidine therapy.

# Disturbances in Atrioventricular Conduction & Atrioventricular Dissociation | 12

## ATRIOVENTRICULAR CONDUCTION DISTURBANCES

Atrioventricular (AV) conduction delay ("block") is a disturbance in conduction of sinus (or atrial) impulses to the ventricles. The more common causes of AV block are listed in Table 12–1.

### First-Degree AV "Block"

First-degree AV block indicates a conduction delay between the atria and the ventricles; all atrial impulses are conducted. It is characterized by a long PR interval, which exceeds 0.20 s (Fig 12–1). The components of the PR interval are interatrial conduction (10–50 ms), AV nodal conduction (90–150 ms), and His-Purkinje conduction (25–55 ms). (SA depolarization occurs prior to the inscription of the P wave and is not recorded on the surface ECG.) The prolonged PR interval of first-degree AV block can therefore reflect prolonged interatrial, intra–AV nodal, or His-Purkinje conduction; it usually represents delay in AV nodal conduction.

**Table 12–1.** Common causes of AV conduction disturbances.

Hypervagotonia (often associated with sinus bradycardia or sinus arrhythmia)
Digitalis
Beta-blocking drugs
Some calcium channel–blocking drugs (verapamil, diltiazem)
Coronary artery disease
   Inferior wall myocardial infarction (AV nodal ischemia)
   Right ventricular myocardial infarction (AV nodal ischemia)
   Anterior wall myocardial infarction (interventricular septal necrosis, often associated with bundle branch block)
Lenegre's disease (diffuse fibrosis of the conduction system)
Infiltrative heart disease
Calcification of the mitral anulus
Acute infectious diseases
Myocarditis

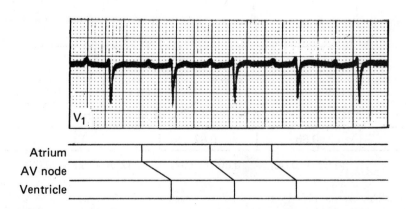

**Figure 12–1.** First-degree AV block. The PR interval is prolonged to 0.28 s. The laddergram beneath the ECG illustrates the 3 levels of AV conduction: the atrium, the AV node, and the ventricles, with the delay in AV conduction occurring in the AV node.

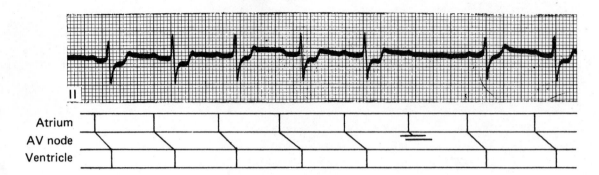

**Figure 12–2.** Type I (Wenckebach) second-degree AV block in which the sinus impulse is conducted to the ventricles with progressive delay (progressively increasing PR intervals) until an impulse fails to be conducted. Although type I AV block can occur in the His-Purkinje system, it most commonly represents AV nodal conduction delay, as illustrated in the laddergram.

## Second-Degree AV "Block"

Second-degree AV block describes a situation in which not all atrial impulses are conducted to the ventricles. Type I (Wenckebach) second-degree AV block is present when atrial impulses encounter progressive delay in conduction to the ventricles because of AV nodal refractoriness, with eventual failure of conduction of an impulse (Fig 12–2). The ratio of P waves to QRS complexes is used to describe the AV conduction ratio in type I second-degree AV block and may thus be 4:3, 8:7, etc. This ratio is also referred to as a **Wenckebach period.** Because type I second-degree AV block usually occurs within the AV node, the PR interval of the first conducted P wave of the Wenckebach period is often prolonged. And, because this form of conduction disturbance involves the AV node rather than the bundle branches, the QRS complexes are usually narrow and appear normal.

The Wenckebach period may be described as follows (Fig 12–3). The sinus rate is constant. As the sinus impulses are conducted through the AV node, they encounter increasing conduction delay (prolongation of PR intervals). However, the *increment* in conduction delay from one P–QRS complex to the next is slightly less each time, resulting in a shortening of the RR interval relative to the preceding RR interval. Finally, a P wave fails to be conducted. The RR interval encompassing the nonconducted P wave is twice the PP interval *minus* the total increment in the PR intervals of the Wenckebach period. In a typical or classic Wenckebach period, therefore, 3 "rules" obtain: (1) the PR intervals progressively lengthen; (2) the RR intervals progressively shorten; and (3) the RR interval encompassing the nonconducted P wave is less than twice the preceding RR interval. Whereas typical Wenckebach periods are usually seen with low AV

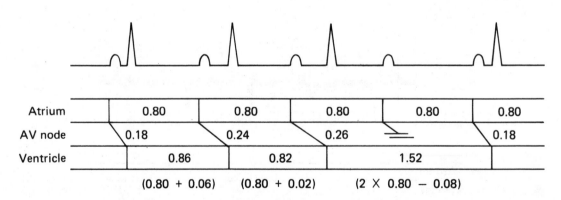

**Figure 12–3.** A typical Wenckebach period with a 4:3 AV conduction ratio (four P waves and three QRS complexes). The sinus cycle length is constant at 0.80 s. The PR intervals progressively increase from 0.18 to 0.24 to 0.26 s; however, the *increment* in increase in PR intervals is 0.06 s between the first and second PR intervals and 0.02 s between the second and third PR intervals. Thus, the increment in PR interval increase is less each time. The RR cycle lengths equal the PP cycle lengths plus the increment in PR interval; thus, the RR cycle lengths get progressively shorter. The RR interval encompassing the nonconducted P wave is twice the sinus cycle length less the *total* increment in all PR intervals during the Wenckebach period.

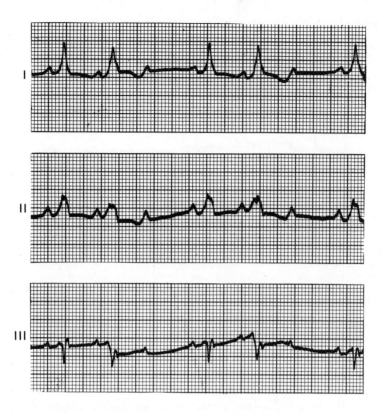

**Figure 12–4.** Type II (Mobitz II) second-degree AV block, with a 3:2 AV conduction ratio. The atrial rhythm is sinus. The PR intervals of the conducted beats are normal and constant. Every third P wave fails to be conducted to the ventricles. In addition to the AV block, left bundle branch block is present, with the second of each set of QRS complexes being more aberrant than the first. This suggests a progressive degree of conduction delay in the left bundle branch itself, that is, Wenckebach type block in the left bundle branch.

conduction ratios (3:2, 4:3, or 5:4), as the AV conduction ratio increases (exceeding 6:5), more Wenckebach sequences are atypical and do not follow the classic rules.

Type II (Mobitz II) second-degree AV block is present when atrial impulses fail to be transmitted to the ventricles without prior progressive conduction delay. Thus, failure of antegrade conduction is often abrupt and unpredictable. In contrast to type I second-degree AV block, in which the conduction delay is in the AV node, the conduction block in type II second-degree AV block may be within the bundle of His or, more commonly, distal to the bundle of His in the bundle branches. Therefore, the QRS complexes often show a bundle branch block pattern, and the PR interval of the conducted P waves is constant and often normal (Fig 12–4).

### 2:1 AV Block

Second-degree AV block with a 2:1 AV conduction ratio may represent either type I (Wenckebach) or type II (Mobitz II) second-degree AV block (Fig 12–5). Since 2 consecutive PR intervals are not recorded, the differential diagnosis may be dif-

ficult. However, certain general rules apply. If the PR interval of the conducted P waves is prolonged and the QRS complexes are narrow and appear normal, type I AV block (intra–AV nodal) is probably present. If the PR interval of the conducted P waves is normal and the QRS complexes show a bundle branch block pattern, type II AV block (distal to the bundle of His) is probably present. If the PR interval of the conducted P wave is prolonged and the QRS complexes show a bundle branch block pattern, or if the PR interval of the conducted P wave is normal and the QRS complexes appear normal, it may be impossible to distinguish between type I and type II second-degree AV block. Changing the AV conduction ratio from 2:1 to 3:2 or more by means of carotid sinus massage or intravenous atropine will often unmask the nature and therefore the location of the AV block.

### Complete (High-Grade) AV "Block"

In complete AV block, the atria and ventricles are depolarized independently of each other (Figs 12–6 and 12–7). Because of the high degree of AV

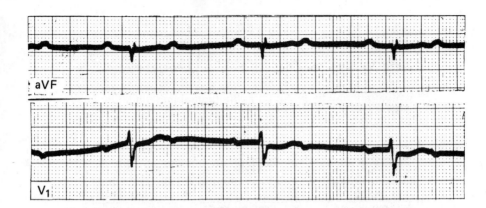

**Figure 12–5.** AV block with a 2:1 AV conduction ratio. The PR interval of the conducted P waves is prolonged, and the QRS complexes are narrow and appear normal. (The Q wave in aVF suggests inferior wall myocardial infarction.) When the conduction ratio is 2:1, it is often not possible to tell with certainty whether the block is in the AV node or in the His-Purkinje system. A change in the AV conduction ratio with a consequent demonstration of Wenckebach periodicity or type II block would be required for the precise diagnosis. However, 2:1 AV block in which the QRS complexes are of normal duration and the PR interval of the conducted beats is prolonged is usually occurring within the AV node; whereas 2:1 AV block in which the QRS complexes show a bundle branch block pattern and the PR interval of the conducted beats is normal often indicates a block below the level of the AV node.

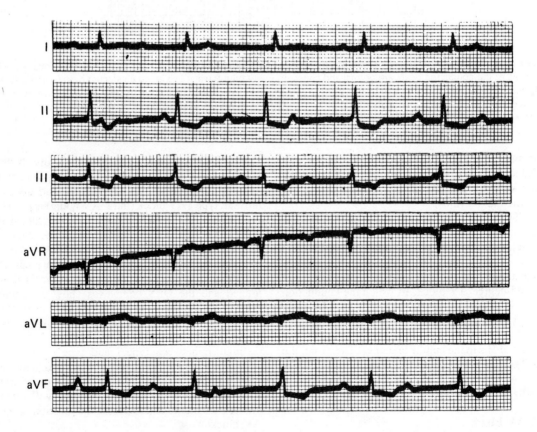

**Figure 12–6.** Complete AV block. The atrial rhythm is regular at a rate of 82/min. The ventricular rhythm is regular at a rate of 60/min. There is no relation between the 2 rhythms; the atria respond to the sinus node and the ventricles respond to an independent pacemaker. Since the QRS complexes are of normal duration and configuration, the ventricular pacemaker is likely to be originating in the AV junction or bundle of His. The apparent widening of some of the QRS complexes (fifth QRS in lead III and third QRS in lead aVF) is the result of fortuitous superimposition of the P wave upon the QRS complex.

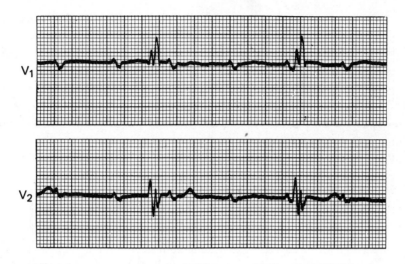

**Figure 12–7.** Complete AV block. The atrial rhythm is sinus at a rate of 88/min. The ventricular rhythm is regular at a rate of 37/min and is completely independent of the atrial rhythm. The QRS complexes are wide and show a right bundle branch block pattern. The long QRS duration and the slow rate of the QRS rhythm suggest a ventricular focus of origin.

block, no atrial impulse can be conducted to the ventricles despite temporal opportunity to do so. Temporal opportunity is a term used to describe a particular set of electrophysiologic conditions that must be present in order to allow transmission of the atrial impulse through the AV node–His–Purkinje system. The atrial rate in complete AV block is almost always faster than the ventricular rate. The ventricular pacemaker originates distal to the site of block and may be in the AV junction, bundle of His, bundle branches, or distal Purkinje system. In complete AV block, the QRS rhythm is an **escape rhythm;** the morphology of the complexes and their rate will depend upon the site of origin.

### Vagotonic Block

A high degree of vagal tone, such as occurs with sympathetic withdrawal during sleep, may be associated with (1) slowing of sinus rate; (2) pauses in sinus rhythm; (3) variable degrees of delay in AV conduction, manifested by (often irregular) prolongation of the PR interval; and (4) failure of conduction of P waves in a manner resembling type I (Wenckebach) or even type II AV block (Fig 12–8). It is important to recognize vagotonic block, since it often occurs in normal individuals as well as in patients with inferior or right ventricular myocardial infarction (or both) or any other clinical condition in which hypervagotonia is present. It not uncommonly accompanies the use of certain medications, notably beta-adrenergic blocking agents and antihypertensive drugs.

## ATRIOVENTRICULAR DISSOCIATION

AV dissociation is present when one pacemaker activates the atria and a second independent pacemaker activates the ventricles. The atrial pacemaker is usually the sinus node, but any atrial rhythm can be present. The ventricular pacemaker can originate in the AV junction, bundle of His, bundle branches, or peripheral Purkinje tissue. Its rate is usually faster than that of the atria. When the 2 rates are about the same, resulting in apparent association of atrial and ventricular rhythms, the AV dissociation is termed **isorhythmic.** If the atrial rhythm is an ectopic tachycardia and the ventricular rhythm represents acceleration of a subsidiary pacemaker, **double tachycardia** is said to be present. Emergence of the ventricular pacemaker can come about as a result of acceleration of the rate of the subsidiary pacemaker because of enhanced automaticity (**accelerated rhythm**) (Fig 12–9) or as a result of slowing of the atrial rate below the intrinsic rate of the lower pacemaker, which will then take over as an **escape rhythm.**

AV dissociation is not a form of complete AV block. In AV block, atrial impulses *cannot* be conducted to the ventricles despite temporal opportunity for this to occur. In contrast, in AV dissociation, atrial impulses will *capture* (be conducted to and stimulate) the ventricles if temporal opportunity is provided. Long rhythm strips must sometimes be recorded in order to demonstrate the presence of capture, which is the hallmark of AV dissociation (Fig 12–9).

Continuous recording

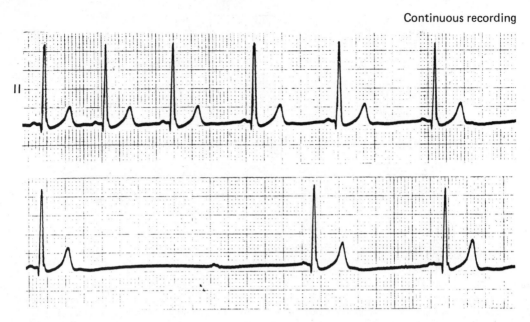

**Figure 12–8.** Vagotonic block in a young postoperative herniorrhaphy patient, recorded during sleep. The atrial rhythm is sinus. Slowing of the sinus rhythm occurs gradually, eventuating in a pause of almost 2 s. This pause is accompanied by failure of conduction of the P wave to the ventricles. Following the pause, sinus rhythm with normal AV conduction is again present. Vagotonic AV block should not be confused with type I or type II AV block. The diagnosis depends upon the demonstration of slowing of the sinus rate in association with failure of AV conduction, if present.

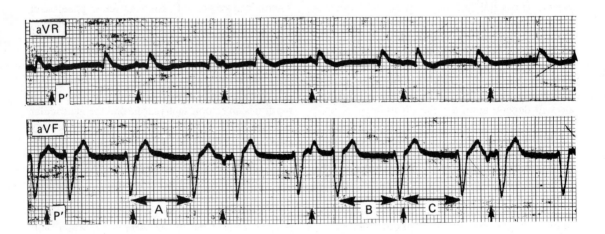

**Figure 12–9.** AV dissociation with capture. Two rhythms are present. A regular atrial rhythm (arrows) is present at a rate of 60/min. The P' waves are upright in aVR and inverted in lead aVF, indicating retrograde atrial activation, presumably from a focus low in the atrium. The QRS rhythm occurs at a rate of 85/min (determined from the RR interval shown at (A), (B), and (C). The rate of the QRS rhythm and the normal duration of the QRS complexes indicate a focus of origin in the AV junction or bundle of His. In aVF, the second, fifth, seventh, and tenth QRS complexes occur early relative to the prevailing QRS rate and are preceded by P' waves at intervals of 0.12 s. These early QRS complexes represent *capture* beats, that is, they are stimulated by the P' waves that precede them. Ventricular capture is the hallmark of AV dissociation.

## TEST TRACINGS

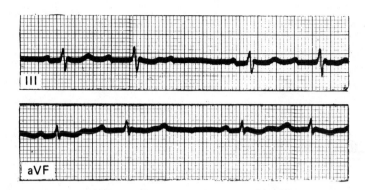

**Figure 12–T1.** Second-degree AV block of the Wenckebach type. The atrial rhythm is regular. In lead III, the first PR interval is 0.18 s, the second 0.28 s, and the third 0.36 s. The third impulse beat fails to activate the ventricle; thus, this is a 3:2 Wenckebach period.

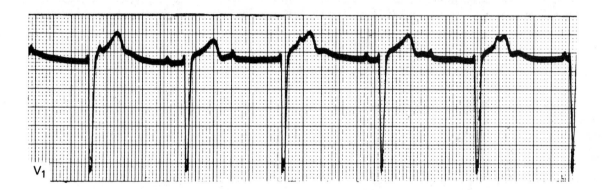

**Figure 12–T2.** Complete AV block. The atrial rhythm is sinus at a rate of 72/min. No P waves are conducted to the ventricles. The ventricular rhythm is regular at a rate of 54/min. Since the QRS complexes are narrow and appear normal, the ventricular pacemaker is probably arising in the AV junction or bundle of His.

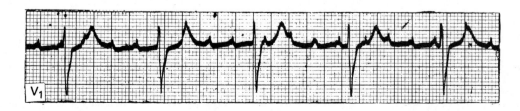

**Figure 12–T3.** Atrial tachycardia with complete AV block. The atrial rate is 230/min. The ventricular rate is regular at 55/min. Since there is no relation between the atrial and ventricular rhythms, complete AV block is present. The rate of the ventricular rhythm and the narrow, relatively normal-appearing QRS complexes suggest that the origin of the ventricular rhythm is the AV junction or the bundle of His.

# 13 | The Ventricular Arrhythmias

## VENTRICULAR PREMATURE COMPLEXES

Ventricular premature complexes can arise from an ectopic focus in any portion of the ventricular myocardium or from reentry of an impulse (ventricular or supraventricular) into and through an area of ventricular tissue (Fig 13–1). When ventricular premature complexes are due to reentry, the impulse conducted into the site of reentry is blocked in one area of ventricular tissue because of refractoriness but is conducted through another area with some delay. The impulse can then turn around and, because of its previously delayed transmission, reexcite the area that was previously refractory, resulting in a reentry beat. Premature ventricular complexes that have a **fixed coupling interval** to the QRS complexes preceding them are thought to arise by this mechanism.

Ventricular premature complexes may be conducted in retrograde fashion into the His bundle and AV node, delaying antegrade conduction of the next sinus beat. They may be conducted to the atria and depolarize the atria in retrograde manner, resulting in an inverted P wave in II, III, and aVF. They may invade the sinus node, depolarize it, and reset its

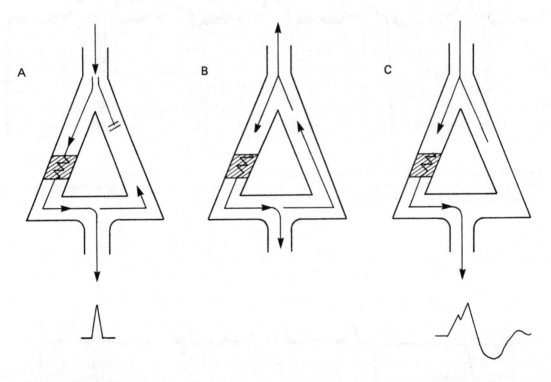

**Figure 13–1.** Reentry as a cause of ventricular extrasystoles. *A:* An impulse (supraventricular or ventricular) conducted from above into an area of ventricular tissue is blocked in one pathway and conducted with delay through another pathway (hatched area). The conducted impulse depolarizes myocardial tissue and also turns around and is conducted in a retrograde direction. *B:* The impulse has conducted in retrograde fashion through the area previously refractory and turns in antegrade fashion. *C:* The same impulse has again propagated through the area of conduction delay to the surrounding myocardium, in a particular temporal relationship to the original impulse (**coupled extrasystole**).

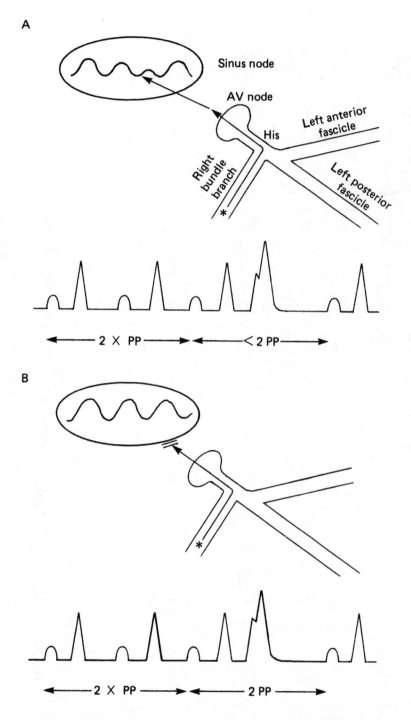

**Figure 13–2.** *A:* The premature ventricular impulse (*) is conducted in retrograde fashion to the atrium and through the SA area, depolarizing the sinus node and resetting its timing. (The partial premature depolarization of the sinus node does not result in atrial activation because of the suboptimal quality of the action potential.) The pause following the ventricular extrasystole is less than fully compensatory, as the PP interval encompassing the premature ventricular complex is less than twice the usual PP interval. *B:* The premature impulse has depolarized the atria in retrograde fashion but has not penetrated the SA area *(entrance block);* thus, the firing rate of the sinus node is not disturbed and the next sinus impulse occurs on time. The PP interval encompassing the premature ventricular complex is twice the normal PP interval, and the pause is fully compensatory.

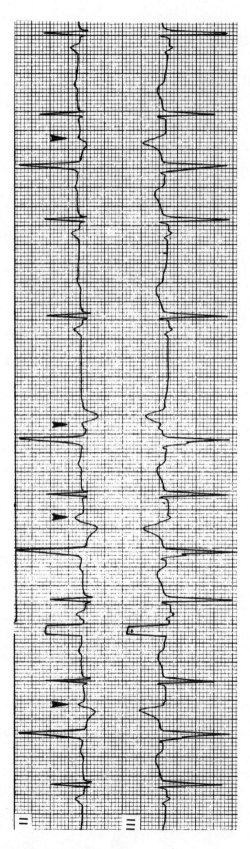

**Figure 13–3.**  Pseudo–AV block due to concealed conduction. Sinus rhythm is present. Frequent uniform premature ventricular complexes are present. The P waves that follow them (arrows) are conducted to the ventricles with first-degree AV block (first, second, and fourth arrows) and are sometimes not conducted at all (third arrow). The AV block is due to concealed retrograde conduction into the AV node of the ventricular premature impulse, delaying or blocking subsequent antegrade impulse conduction.

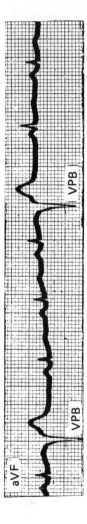

**Figure 13–4.**  Uniform ("monomorphic") premature ventricular complexes. These may arise from a single focus of origin or result from a reentry phenomenon. There is a fixed coupling interval between the sinus beats and the premature ventricular complexes, favoring the latter mechanism. VPB, ventricular premature beats.

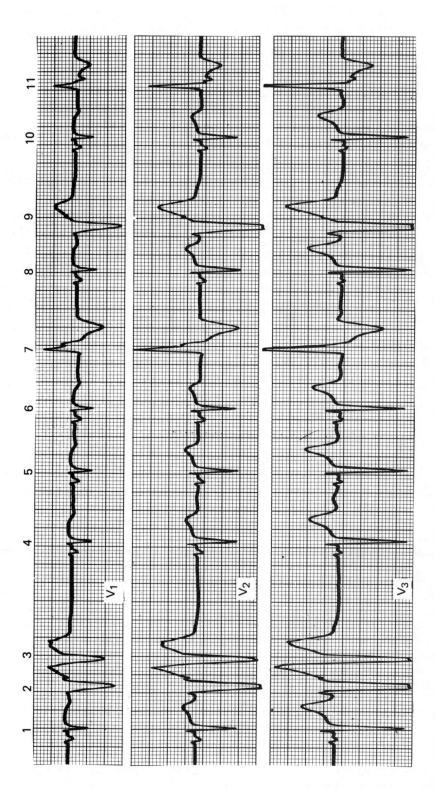

**Figure 13–5.** Multiform premature ventricular complexes. QRS complexes 2, 3, and 9 are oriented posteriorly (deep S waves in $V_{1-3}$), suggesting a right ventricular focus of origin. QRS complexes 7 and 11 are oriented anteriorly (tall R waves in $V_{1-3}$) and suggest a left ventricular focus of origin. However, the site of origin of the ventricular complexes is difficult to tell with certainty, since the QRS configuration reflects intramyocardial impulse conduction and epicardial activation pattern rather than focus locations.

timing, or they may depolarize the atria but not penetrate the sinus node and therefore not reset its timing (Fig 13–2). If the sinus node has been penetrated and reset by the ventricular premature impulse, the interval between the sinus beats enclosing the premature ventricular complex will be less than twice the sinus rate (**less than fully compensatory pause**). If the sinus node is not reset and the sinus firing rate is not disturbed, the next sinus impulse will occur on time. Thus, the interval between the sinus beats enclosing the ventricular premature complex will be twice the sinus rate (**fully compensatory pause**) (Fig 13–2).

Retrograde invasion of the AV node by a ventricular premature impulse can result in delay in antegrade transmission of the next sinus impulse or total failure of conduction of the impulse. Because the retrograde invasion of the AV node is not itself visible on the ECG but is recognized by its effect on subsequent electrocardiographic events, the phenomenon is known as **concealed conduction.** Delay in (or failure of) antegrade AV conduction due to concealed retrograde conduction of a ventricular premature impulse is called **pseudo-AV block** (Fig 13–3).

Premature ventricular complexes may have similar configurations in a given electrocardiographic lead or more than one configuration. Uniform ("monomorphic") premature ventricular complexes may arise from a single focus or result from a reentry pathway (Fig 13–4). Premature ventricular complexes of varying configurations may arise from multiple foci (**multifocal**) or, more commonly, from a single focus but may be conducted through different pathways to depolarize the ventricular myocardium, resulting in different QRS configurations (Fig 13–5). The term **multiform** ("polymorphic" or "multimorphic"), rather than **multifocal,** is therefore more precise in describing premature ventricular complexes of varying configurations.

Ventricular complexes are broad and bizarre in appearance and usually exceed 0.12 s in duration. They are often notched and slurred. The ST segment and T wave are usually displaced in a direction opposite to the main QRS deflection. If a P wave is associated with a premature ventricular complex, it may be a sinus P wave occurring in a fortuitous relation to the ventricular complex and therefore dissociated from it; or it may be a P' wave caused by retrograde activation of the atria by the ventricular impulse (Fig 13–6). The retrograde P' wave will be inverted in II, III, and aVF, and its earlier occurrence in relation to the underlying sinus rate will distinguish it from a sinus impulse.

Occasionally, a premature ventricular complex will occur between 2 sinus impulses without disturbing the sinus rate. This is called an **inter-**

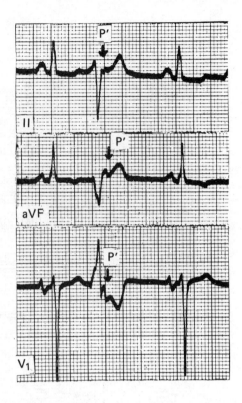

**Figure 13–6.** Premature ventricular complexes. The complexes are broad, bizarre, and prolonged. They are followed by P' waves that are inverted in II and aVF, indicating retrograde atrial activation.

**polated premature ventricular complex** (Fig 13–7).

### R-on-T Premature Ventricular Complexes

Since the QT interval approximates the refractory period of ventricular tissue, a premature ventricular complex is usually inscribed after the T wave of the preceding beat. However, a premature ventricular complex will occasionally begin at the peak of the T wave or on its downstroke (Fig 13–8). R-on-T premature ventricular complexes may fall in the vulnerable period of ventricular tissue, initiating repetitive ventricular beating (tachycardia or fibrillation); they are thus considered to be of serious clinical significance (Fig 13–9).

### Ventricular Bigeminy

In ventricular bigeminy, the rhythm alternates between a sinus beat (or any basic rhythm) and a ventricular premature complex (Fig 13–10). There is usually a constant interval between the sinus and ventricular complexes (**fixed coupling**), suggesting that reentry is the underlying mechanism for the ventricular impulse (Fig 13–1). Ventricular bigeminy is not itself a more dangerous rhythm than isolated premature ventricular beats; the signifi-

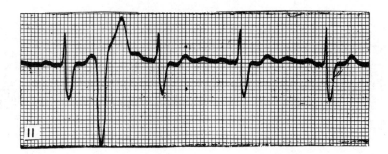

**Figure 13–7.** Interpolated premature ventricular complex. A broad, bizarre premature ventricular complex follows the first sinus-stimulated QRS complex but does not disturb the sinus rate. Thus, the premature ventricular beat is interpolated. The PR intervals of the first, third, and fourth sinus beats are 0.19 s, but that of the second sinus beat is 0.23 s. The prolongation in PR interval following the premature ventricular complex results from concealed retrograde conduction into the AV node by the premature complex, causing subsequent antegrade conduction delay. Note the prominent U waves following the T waves.

aVF

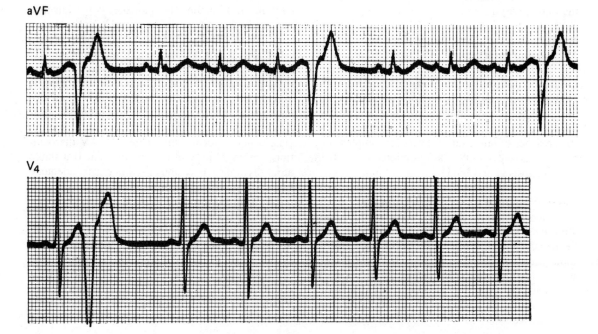

V₄

**Figure 13–8.** R-on-T premature ventricular complexes. The premature complexes are occurring near the peak of the T wave, during the time when the ventricles might be vulnerable to tachycardia or fibrillation. Since not all R-on-T premature ventricular impulses cause ventricular fibrillation, the vulnerable period must occupy an extremely critical time period during repolarization.

I

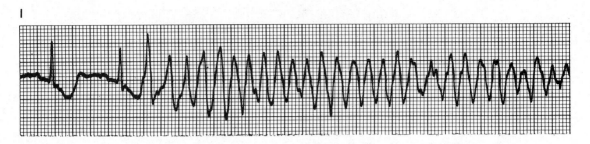

**Figure 13–9.** R-on-T premature ventricular complex occurring at the peak of the T wave of the preceding sinus beat. This premature complex falls during the vulnerable period of the ventricular tissue, resulting in ventricular fibrillation.

cance of the arrhythmia will depend upon the underlying heart disease, if present. Ventricular trigeminy (or quadrigeminy) describes an arrhythmia in which 2 (or 3) sinus beats are followed by a premature ventricular complex in repetitive fashion or in which one sinus beat is followed by 2 (or 3) consecutive premature ventricular complexes in repetitive fashion. Again, the prognosis depends on the underlying disease.

### Premature Ventricular Complexes in Myocardial Infarction

In the presence of myocardial infarction, ventricular premature complexes may show some of the typical features of the infarction pattern, specifically a QR pattern. When myocardial infarction cannot be diagnosed, as in left bundle branch block, the presence of premature ventricular complexes of QR or QRs (but not QS) configuration may confirm the diagnosis (Fig 13–11).

### Postextrasystolic ST–T Wave Changes

Occasionally, the ST–T wave of the sinus-stimulated QRS complex that follows a premature ventricular impulse will be different from that of other sinus-conducted beats (Fig 13–12). Although this postextrasystolic ST–T wave change is commonly seen in patients with coronary artery disease, it is a nonspecific finding and therefore of no clinical significance.

## VENTRICULAR TACHYCARDIA

Ventricular tachycardia is a sustained or non-sustained arrhythmia originating in ventricular tissue, either from an automatic focus, from a reentry pathway, or by triggered automaticity (see Chapter 11). It may occur only within the ventricular myocardium, or it may involve the bundle branches and even the His bundle. Its rate exceeds the intrinsic ventricular rate of 20–50/min and usually ranges from 120 to 220/min. The rhythm may be irregular, especially if the tachycardia is short-lived. Although ventricular tachycardia is always a serious rhythm disturbance that requires early attention, it may or may not be associated with symptoms depending upon the rate of the tachycardia, the relation of ventricular rhythm to atrial rhythm, and the state of the myocardium. If there is AV dissociation, any atrial rhythm may be present. If a stable atrial rhythm such as sinus rhythm exists, adequate filling of the ventricles may occur and cardiac output will be maintained. However, if there is AV association (as in ventriculoatrial conduction), ventricular and atrial systole may occur together, with insufficient time for ventricular filling via atrial systole to occur. Stroke output will fall rapidly, and cerebral hypoperfusion will result. Ventriculoatrial conduction may occur in a 1:1 relationship, a ventriculoatrial Wenckebach type of second-degree block, or a fixed ventriculoatrial block with 2:1 and

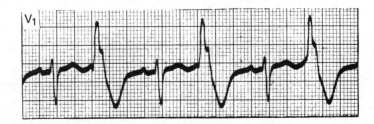

**Figure 13–10.** Ventricular bigeminy. After each sinus-conducted beat, a premature ventricular complex occurs at a fixed coupling interval. The sinus rhythm is undisturbed; however, in this arrhythmia the sinus *rate* cannot be ascertained, since consecutive sinus beats are not present.

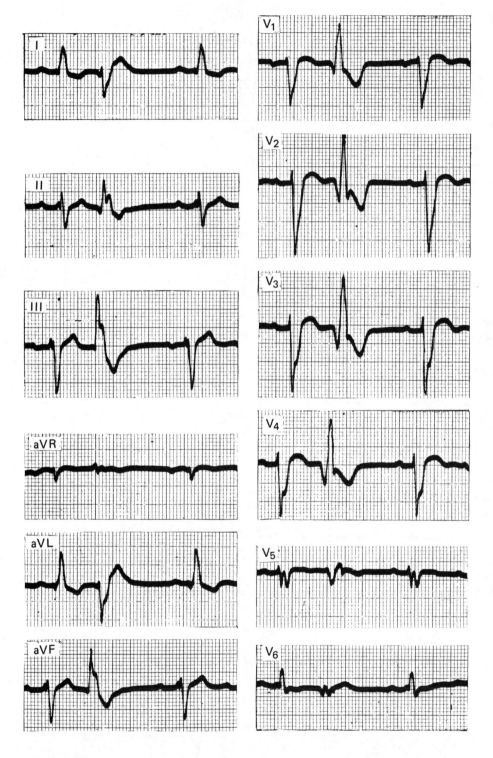

**Figure 13–11.** Premature ventricular complexes occurring in a patient with left bundle branch block pattern. The first and third complexes in each strip are sinus-stimulated, and the second QRS complex is a premature ventricular complex. The left bundle branch block pattern precludes the electrocardiographic diagnosis of myocardial infarction. However, the premature ventricular complexes have a QR pattern in the precordial leads, revealing underlying myocardial infarction (confirmed at autopsy).

Continuous recording

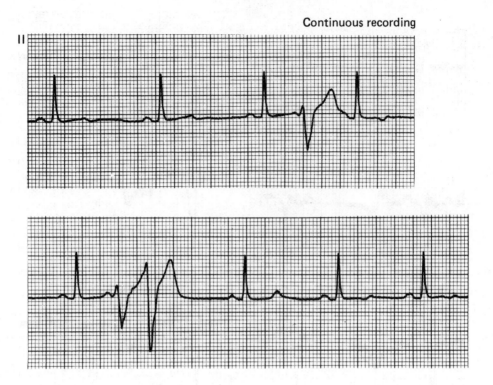

**Figure 13–12.** Postextrasystolic T wave alterations in a healthy 32-year-old man. The postextrasystolic T wave changes are themselves variable. Although this phenomenon was once thought to indicate coronary artery disease, it is now recognized to occur in normal individuals.

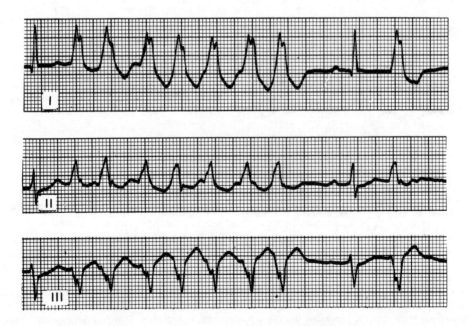

**Figure 13–13.** Sinus rhythm with a burst of ventricular tachycardia. Following the first sinus beat, there are 7 consecutive wide complexes occurring at a slightly irregular rate of 150/min. Following the burst of wide complex tachycardia, a premature ventricular complex is coupled to a sinus complex. Since the configuration of the premature ventricular complex is identical to the tachycardia complexes, the tachycardia is ventricular in origin.

3:1 conduction ratios. Complete ventriculoatrial block may also occur.

Ventricular tachycardia complexes are broad and bizarre and resemble ventricular premature beats (Fig 13–13). The rate is often so rapid that the ST segment and T waves cannot be distinguished from the QRS complexes, and the ECG has the appearance of a series of wide, large undulations. If the atrial rhythm can be identified and AV dissociation demonstrated, the diagnosis of the wide complex tachycardia is ventricular tachycardia until proved otherwise (Fig 13–14).

Ventricular tachycardia may be **bradycardia-dependent,** ie, it may follow a pause in QRS rhythm; the pause may be due to SA block, sinus arrest, or AV block. Bradycardia-dependent ventricular tachycardia is thought to result from a premature ventricular impulse occurring during heterogeneous depolarization-repolarization times in the ventricular myocardium. The heterogeneity in turn results from absence of a stimulus that would normally depolarize the tissue uniformly.

**Bidirectional ventricular tachycardia** is the term applied to a rare form of ventricular tachycardia in which the QRS complexes in any one lead alternate in opposite directions (Fig 13–15).

The electrocardiographic appearance of ventricular tachycardia is variable. Classic patterns have a superior mean frontal plane QRS axis, a qR, QR, or pure R wave configuration in $V_1$, and an rS or QS configuration in $V_6$ (Fig 13–16). Although tachycardias originating in the right ventricle are expected to have the configuration of left bundle branch block (since the right ventricular myocardium is activated in advance of the left ventricular myocardium) and those originating in the left ventricle are expected to have the configuration of right bundle branch block, electrode mapping studies of the endocardium and epicardium indicate that the tachycardia configuration does not necessarily indicate its origin. Whereas tachycardias with a right

bundle branch block pattern often do originate in the left ventricular myocardium, most of those with a left bundle branch block pattern also originate in the left ventricular myocardium, particularly in the paraseptal area.

On occasion, the QRS configuration of ventricular tachycardia can vary; the arrhythmia is then termed **polymorphic ventricular tachycardia.** Changes in QRS configuration do not indicate different foci of origin of impulses but rather reflect different pathways of myocardial activation taken by the tachycardia impulses.

A particular type of polymorphic ventricular tachycardia, in which the QRS complex configurations appear to undulate around an isoelectric baseline, is known as **torsade de pointes** (Fig 13–17). This form of ventricular tachycardia is most often seen in the presence of a long QTU interval due to any cause and may result from disparate depolarization-repolarization times in His-Purkinje tissue, reflected in the long QTU interval. The tachycardia often occurs in self-terminating bursts but can degenerate into ventricular fibrillation.

## DIFFERENTIATION OF VENTRICULAR TACHYCARDIA FROM SUPRAVENTRICULAR TACHYCARDIA WITH INTRAVENTRICULAR ABERRATION

The differential diagnosis of ventricular tachycardia from supraventricular tachycardia with intraventricular aberration can be difficult (see Chapter 14). If the atrial rhythm is fibrillation, the gross irregularity of the ventricular rhythm indicates that the QRS complexes are stimulated by the atrial fibrillation (Fig 13–18).

If the atrial rhythm is sinus, it will occur at a rate independent from that of the ventricular

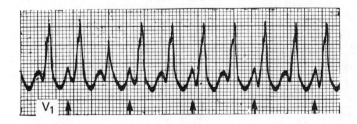

**Figure 13–14.** Ventricular tachycardia with AV dissociation. A wide complex rhythm is occurring at a rate of 173/min. The complexes have a pure R wave configuration in $V_1$. In alternate ST–T segments sharp deflections occur regularly at a rate of 95/min (arrows) and may be independent of the ventricular rhythm. If so, the atrial rhythm is sinus, the ventricular rhythm is ventricular tachycardia, and AV dissociation is present. An alternate explanation is that the wide complex tachycardia shows 2:1 ventriculoatrial conduction, with retrograde P waves occurring after every second tachycardia complex. Leads II or aVF would be required to ascertain the sequence of atrial depolarization.

V₁                                                                    Continuous recording

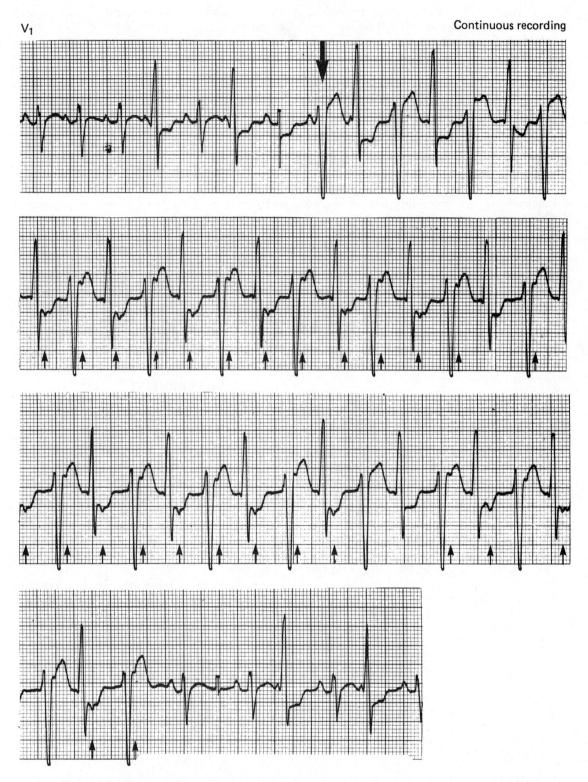

**Figure 13–15.**  Bidirectional ventricular tachycardia in a patient with digitalis toxicity. The first three P–QRS complexes are sinus-stimulated, and the PR interval is 0.16 s. The fourth and sixth complexes are ventricular in origin and are dissociated from the P waves that precede them at short intervals. The third premature ventricular complex (large arrow) initiates a run of wide complex tachycardia with alternation of two QRS configurations. At the beginning of the second strip, 1:1 ventriculoatrial conduction occurs (small arrows). The tachycardia terminates spontaneously, and sinus rhythm resumes.

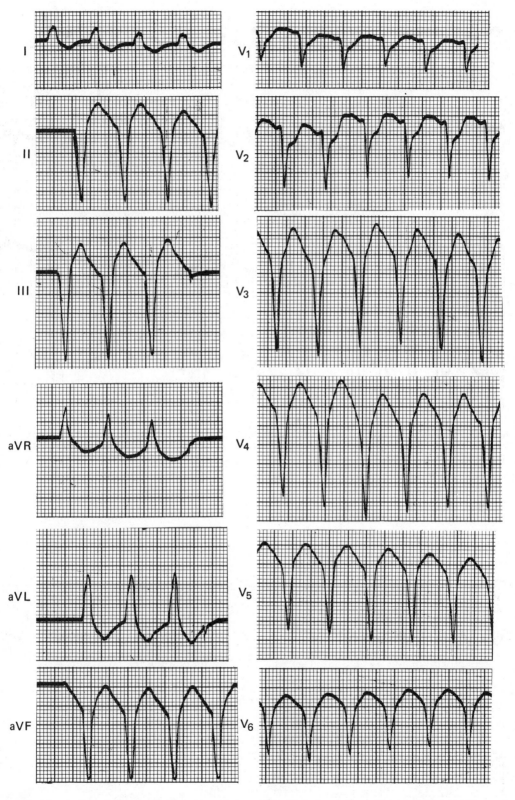

**Figure 13–16.** Ventricular tachycardia. The mean frontal plane QRS axis is directed superiorly and leftward. QS complexes are present in $V_{1-6}$ (*concordance* of QRS complex configuration). Atrial activity is discerned at times (eg, in the T wave of the second QRS complex in $V_2$) and is unrelated to the QRS rhythm.

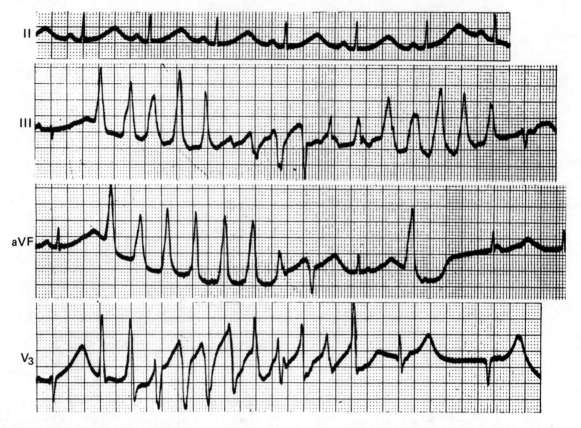

**Figure 13–17.** Polymorphic ventricular tachycardia. Sinus rhythm with a long QT interval is present. Self-terminating bursts of ventricular tachycardia are occurring, in which the QRS configuration is extremely variable and at times appears to rotate about an isoelectric point (**torsade de pointes**).

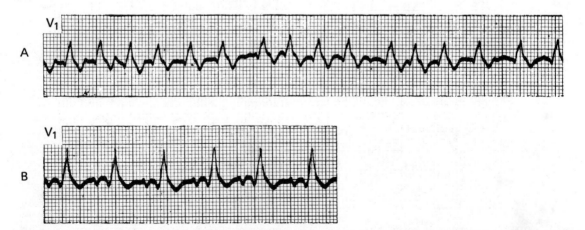

**Figure 13–18.** Atrial fibrillation with intraventricular conduction delay. *A:* Atrial fibrillation with wide complex ventricular rhythm at an irregular rate. The irregularity of the ventricular rhythm is evidence that it is not ventricular tachycardia. *B:* After sinus rhythm is restored, the pattern of intraventricular conduction is seen to be identical to that in (A).

tachycardia and will therefore be dissociated from it. A wide complex tachycardia with AV dissociation is likely to be ventricular in origin. The same principle applies to an automatic atrial tachycardia. The simultaneous occurrence of an automatic atrial tachycardia and a ventricular tachycardia is known as **double tachycardia.**

If the atrial rhythm is flutter, differential diagnosis of a wide complex tachycardia will depend more upon the shape of the QRS complexes and the behavior of the rhythm during maneuvers that delay conduction at the AV node, such as carotid sinus massage. Carotid sinus massage is expected to slow the ventricular rate if the ventricular rhythm is stimulated by the flutter waves; it usually has no effect on ventricular tachycardia.

It may be impossible to distinguish between supraventricular reciprocating tachycardia with aberrant intraventricular conduction and ventricular tachycardia if ventriculoatrial association with 1:1 ventriculoatrial conduction of the tachycardia complexes to the atria is present (Fig 13–19). Again, response to vagal maneuvers may be helpful; increasing AV block by vagal maneuvers is expected to terminate a reciprocating supraventricular tachycardia, whereas no effect on ventricular tachycardia will be observed. Occasionally, vagal maneuvers will produce ventriculoatrial block and alter 1:1 ventriculoatrial conduction to 2:1, Wenckebach, or complete retrograde ventriculoatrial block; this will aid in establishing the diagnosis of ventricular tachycardia.

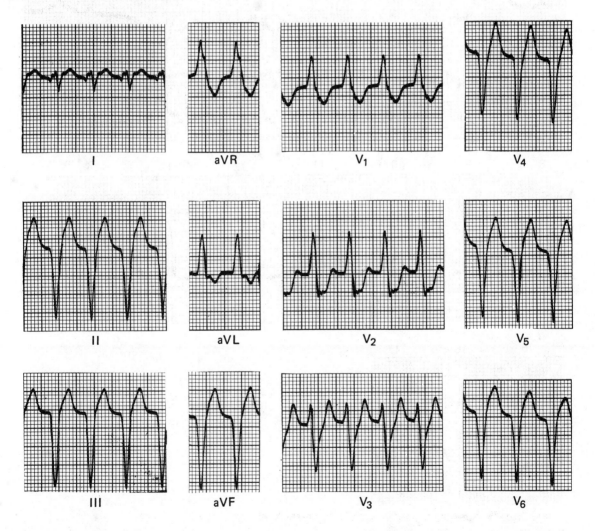

**Figure 13–19.** Wide complex tachycardia, which could be reciprocating supraventricular tachycardia with intraventricular aberration or ventricular tachycardia. The mean frontal plane axis of the tachycardia complexes is superior and rightward, and the precordial lead configuration suggests ventricular tachycardia (pure R wave in $V_1$ and a QS wave in $V_6$). P waves are seen following the QRS complexes in $V_{1-2}$, which, since they could represent either retrograde atrial activation from ventricular tachycardia or reciprocating supraventricular tachycardia, do not help to differentiate between the two. In this case, the configuration of the QRS complexes is the best evidence as to the ventricular origin of the tachycardia.

## ACCELERATED VENTRICULAR RHYTHM

Accelerated ventricular rhythm is a ventricular rhythm that is faster than an "idioventricular" rhythm (usual rate, 30–40/min) but slower than rapid ventricular tachycardia. It is characterized by 3 features: (1) emergence as a result of slight slowing of the sinus rate; (2) disappearance as a result of an increase in the sinus rate; and (3) onset and offset via fusion complexes, in which the ventricles are depolarized by both the sinus impulse and the ventricular focus (Fig 13–20). As this rhythm is considered to be benign, its recognition is most important. Since it is actually an escape rhythm, no treatment is indicated. Accelerated ventricular rhythm must be distinguished from "slow ventricular tachycardia" (Fig 13–21), in which the onset is via a premature ventricular complex without prior fusion and the offset is spontaneous and unrelated to an increase in the sinus rate.

Continuous recording

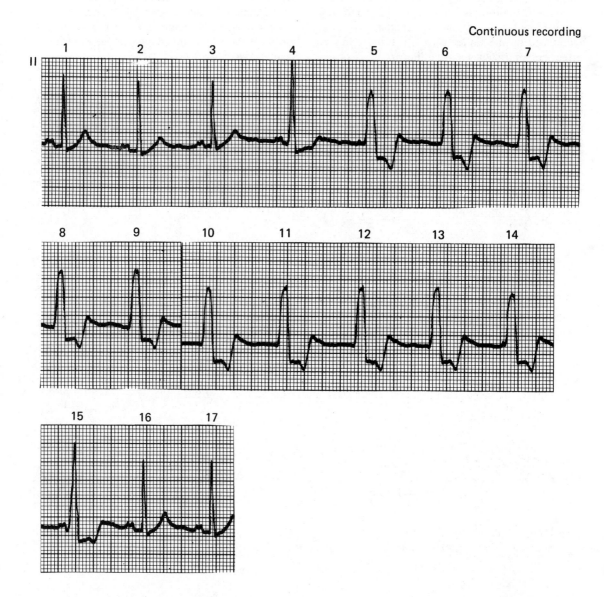

**Figure 13–20.** Accelerated ventricular rhythm. QRS complexes 1, 2, 3, 16, and 17 are sinus-conducted beats. Beats 5 through 14 have wide QRS complexes, are not preceded by P waves, and are regular at a rate of 75/min. Complexes 4 and 15 are preceded by sinus P waves but with shorter PR intervals and longer QRS intervals than the sinus-conducted beats. These are fusion beats, in which ventricular depolarization results in part from the sinus impulse and in part from the ventricular focus. Onset and offset of accelerated ventricular rhythm depends upon the slowing and subsequent increase in the sinus rate, respectively.

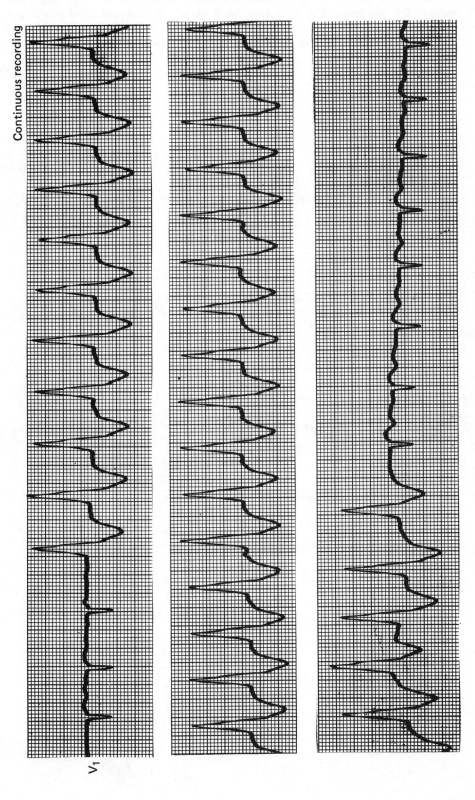

Continuous recording

$V_1$

**Figure 13–21.** "Slow ventricular tachycardia." The rhythm is atrial fibrillation. A self-terminating wide complex rhythm of pure R wave configuration occurs, initially at a rate of about 100/min, and increases to 120/min. The QRS configuration of the wide complex rhythm suggests a ventricular origin; its somewhat irregular rate is not inconsistent with this diagnosis. "Slow ventricular tachycardia" must be distinguished from accelerated ventricular rhythm, as the former is not necessarily benign, whereas the latter more often is.

## VENTRICULAR FIBRILLATION

Ventricular fibrillation is a rapid, irregular, disorganized ventricular rhythm resulting in lack of cardiac output and absent pulse and blood pressure. It results from a premature ventricular complex oc-curring in the vulnerable period of ventricular tissue. The ECG shows bizarre complexes of varying sizes and configurations (Fig 13–22). Electrical defibrillation is the only means of management; otherwise, death will result. Rarely, an episode of ventricular fibrillation is self-terminating.

V₄                                                        Continuous recording

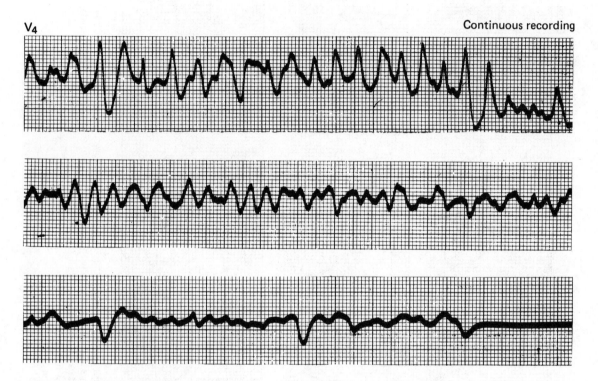

**Figure 13–22.** Ventricular fibrillation. The ventricular complexes are rapid, irregular, and bizarre—typical of ventricular fibrillation. The rhythm terminates with asystole.

## TEST TRACINGS

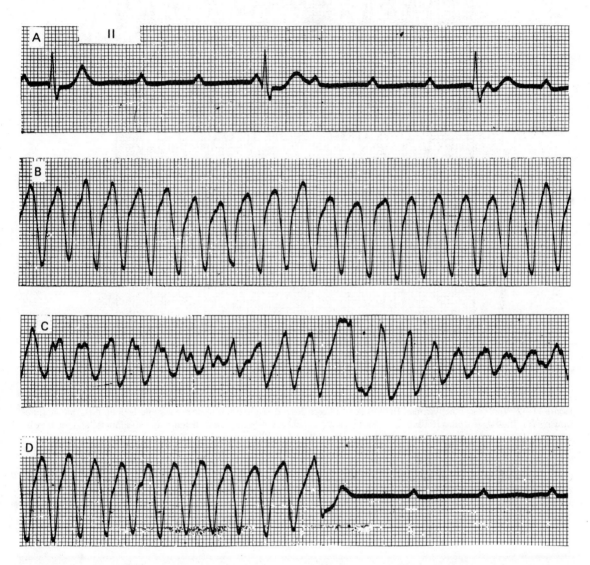

**Figure 13—T1.** Complete AV block with ventricular tachycardia and ventricular asystole. **A:** Complete heart block: The atrial rate is 92/min, and the ventricular rate is 25/min. **B:** Ventricular tachycardia at a rate of 200/min. The QRS complexes are wide, undulating waves. **C:** Ventricular tachycardia-fibrillation. The QRS complexes are more bizarre than in (B) and vary in size and configuration. **D:** Ventricular tachycardia terminating spontaneously, resulting in ventricular asystole. Atrial activity is now seen.

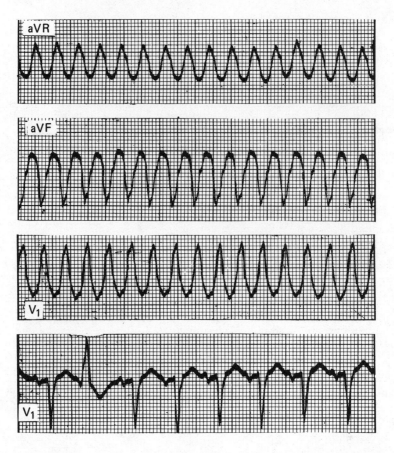

**Figure 13 –T2.** Ventricular tachycardia. The QRS complexes are broad and bizarre and are superiorly directed (QS configuration in aVF). They have a pure R wave configuration in $V_1$. Atrial activity is not clearly discerned, although deflections may be seen following the QRS complexes in aVF and $V_1$. The differential diagnosis includes atrial flutter with 1:1 AV conduction, reciprocating supraventricular tachycardia with intraventricular aberration, and ventricular tachycardia. Sinus rhythm is present in the bottom $V_1$ strip. A single premature complex resembling the tachycardia complexes is recorded; it is preceded by the beginning of a P wave (from which it is dissociated) and has a qR configuration, indicating a ventricular origin. The wide complex tachycardia was therefore ventricular tachycardia.

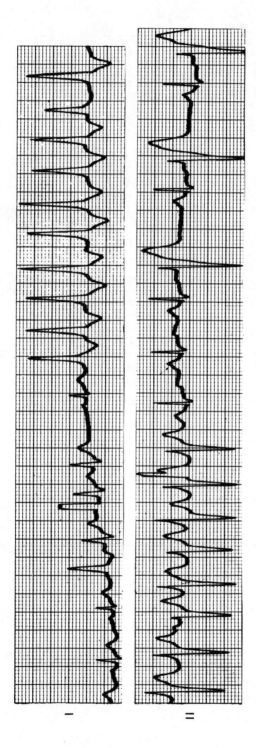

**Figure 13–T3.** Sinus rhythm with bursts of self-terminating ventricular tachycardia. Although the wide QRS complexes resemble a left intraventricular conduction delay, they are not preceded by P waves (except fortuitous sinus P waves), and their rhythm is slightly irregular, indicating a ventricular origin.

**Continuous recording**

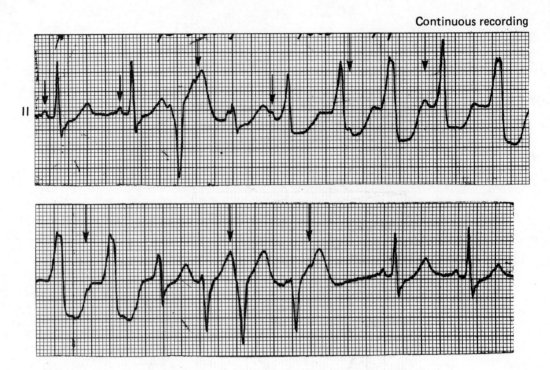

II

**Figure 13—T4.** Slow polymorphic ventricular tachycardia with AV dissociation. Sinus rhythm is present at a regular rate of 74/min. Sinus P waves continue to occur independently of the ventricular tachycardia; thus, AV dissociation is present. A premature ventricular complex (third QRS complex) initiates a 13-beat run of slow ventricular tachycardia of varying QRS configuration. The varying configurations of the tachycardia complexes do not indicate different foci of origin but different pathways of myocardial activation. Hence, the term "multiform" (or "multimorphic") ventricular tachycardia is preferred to "multifocal."

# Aberrancy of Intraventricular Conduction in Association With Supraventricular Arrhythmias | 14

Wide, notched, bizarre QRS complexes may be seen in association with any atrial or AV junctional rhythm and may thus simulate a ventricular arrhythmia. The abnormal QRS configuration may be due to preexisting bundle branch block or ventricular preexcitation (see Chapters 8 and 16), in which case it will be present during sinus rhythm, or it may be seen only during an arrhythmia, with normal intraventricular conduction being present at other times. When atrial activity is seen to precede the abnormal QRS complexes, the diagnosis of intraventricular aberration may easily be made (Fig 14–1). However, when atrial activity is not easily seen to be related to ventricular activity, the differential diagnosis of intraventricular aberration versus ventricular arrhythmia may be difficult (Fig 14–2). Carotid sinus massage may be helpful if the expected AV block is achieved (Fig 14–3) but is not helpful when this response does not occur. Comparison with prior ECGs to establish the presence or absence of intraventricular conduction delay will aid in ascertaining the origin of the QRS complexes. Special leads (intracardiac or esophageal) may clarify the presence and rate of atrial activity but will not aid in determining the relation (antegrade or retrograde) between atrial and ventricular activity if there is one P wave associated with each QRS complex.

An important morphologic feature that favors intraventricular aberration over ventricular ectopy is a right bundle branch block configuration of the premature QRS complexes (Fig 14–4). A right bundle branch block configuration occurs because the right bundle branch normally has the longest refractory period of the intraventricular conduction system (followed in turn by the anterior division of the left bundle branch and the posterior division of the left bundle branch). Thus, premature impulses are more likely to arrive at the right bundle branch when it is still refractory, and their conduction in this bundle branch is therefore more likely to be delayed or blocked.

Another feature of intraventricular aberration is termed the **long-short rule** (Ashman phenomenon). When a QRS complex follows another QRS complex at a given rate (cycle length) and the third QRS has a short coupling interval to the second, the third QRS may show aberrant intraventricular conduction. This occurs because the duration of the refractory period of the bundle branches is related to the heart rate: Slowing the heart rate (increasing the RR cycle length) lengthens the refractory period; thus, if the next impulse is early, it will be blocked in the refractory bundle branch and conducted to the ventricles aberrantly (Fig 14–5). However, since a long RR cycle length also favors the appearance of a

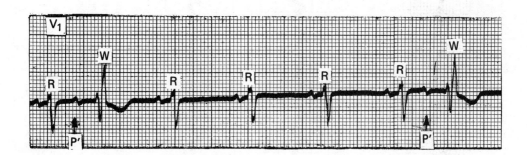

**Figure 14–1.** Premature atrial complexes with aberrant intraventricular conduction. The rhythm is sinus, and the PR interval is 0.16 s. Premature atrial complexes (P') (arrows) are conducted to the ventricles with a PR interval of 0.24 s, reflecting conduction delay in the AV node due to depolarization by the preceding sinus impulse. The QRS complexes stimulated by the P' waves have a right bundle branch block pattern, reflecting refractoriness in this bundle branch at the time of arrival of the premature atrial impulses.

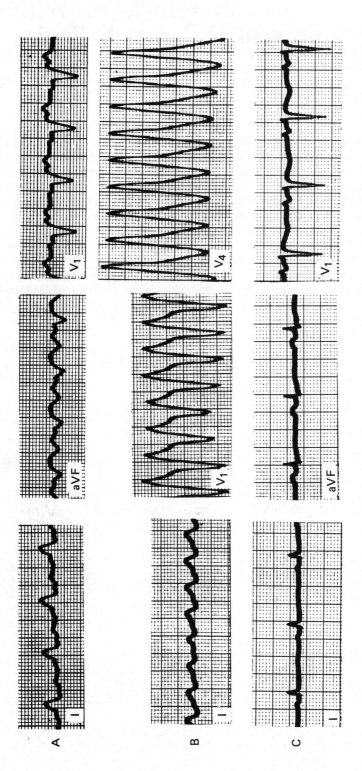

**Figure 14–2.** Automatic atrial tachycardia with changing AV conduction ratios and in-traventricular aberration. *A*: A wide complex tachycardia (rate, 100/min) suggesting left bundle branch block is present; P' waves are occurring at 200/min (best seen in V₁). Thus, the rhythm is atrial tachycardia with 2:1 AV conduction. *B*: Acceleration of the ventricular rate to 200/min as the AV conduction ratio becomes 1:1. The QRS complexes are broader and more bizarre; the rhythm now cannot be distinguished from ventricular tachycardia based on this recording alone. *C*: Restoration of sinus rhythm. The sinus-stimulated QRS complexes resemble the tachycardia complexes except for aberration in the latter complexes (especially noteworthy in aVF). Comparison records are extremely helpful in assessing the origin of wide complex QRS rhythms.

Continuous recording

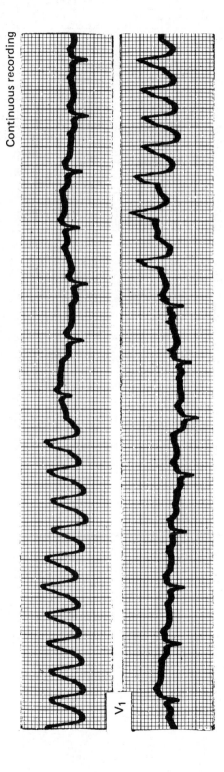

**Figure 14–3.** Effect of carotid sinus massage on a wide QRS complex tachycardia. Broad, bizarre QRS complexes having a pure R wave configuration in $V_1$ occur at a regular rate of 200/min. It is not possible to tell whether this represents ventricular tachycardia or supraventricular tachycardia with intraventricular aberration. Carotid sinus massage results in slowing of the ventricular rate to 100/min and the appearance of a discernible atrial tachycardia (or slow atrial flutter) at a rate of 200/min; thus, 2:1 AV conduction of the atrial impulses has been produced, and the wide complex tachycardia represented intraventricular aberration. Upon cessation of carotid sinus massage, 1:1 AV conduction of the atrial impulses resumes, with reappearance of the wide QRS complexes. This tracing illustrates that intraventricular aberration is often a rate-dependent (tachycardia-dependent) phenomenon.

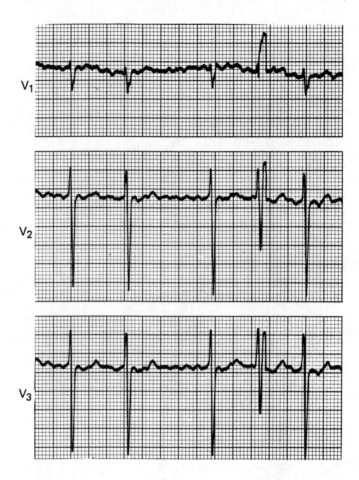

**Figure 14-4.** Atrial fibrillation with aberrant intraventricular conduction. The fourth QRS complex has an rsR' pattern in V$_{1-3}$, indicating right ventricular conduction delay. This complex follows the preceding QRS complex by a short interval, which in turn follows the one preceding it by a longer interval, illustrating the "long-short" rule. Right bundle branch block pattern in an early QRS complex is related to the longer refractory period in the right bundle branch compared to that in the other fascicles and indicates aberrancy of intraventricular conduction.

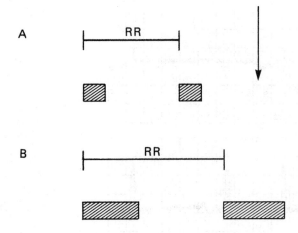

**Figure 14–5.** Schema of the refractory period (hatched areas) of a bundle branch in relation to heart rate (RR cycle length). *A:* At a faster heart rate (shorter RR cycle length) the refractory period is short. An early impulse (arrow) arrives at the bundle branch when it is no longer refractory, and intraventricular conduction is normal. *B:* Slower heart rate (longer RR cycle length) with proportionately longer refractory period of the bundle branches. The premature impulse now arrives during the refractory period of a bundle branch and is not conducted down that bundle branch. Ventricular depolarization will be aberrant.

**Table 14–1.** Features differentiating intraventricular aberration from ventricular ectopy.

| Aberration | Ectopy |
|---|---|
| Preceded by premature P′ wave (unless AV junctional in origin). | Not preceded by premature P′ wave. |
| Triphasic rSR′ in $V_1$; Rs with wide s in $V_6$. | R, RR′, QR in $V_1$; rS or QR in $V_6$. |
| Initial vector of depolarization in $V_1$ the same as during normal intraventricular conduction. | Initial vector of depolarization in $V_1$ opposite to that during normal intraventricular conduction (unless an initial q wave is present). |
| Absence of fixed coupling interval between normally conducted and wide QRS complexes. | Fixed coupling interval between wide QRS complexes and normally conducted complexes. |
| Absence of long interval between wide QRS complex and subsequent QRS complex in atrial fibrillation. | Long interval between wide QRS complex and subsequent normal QRS complex in atrial fibrillation (may not be present). |
| QRS duration often less than 0.14 s. | QRS duration often greater than or equal to 0.14 s. |
| Often resembles a defined bundle branch block pattern. | Superior frontal plane QRS axis. |

premature ventricular complex (**rule of bigeminy),** the long-short rule may not always be helpful in differentiating supraventricular complexes with intraventricular aberration from ectopic ventricular complexes.

Table 14–1 lists those features that help to distinguish intraventricular aberration from ventricular ectopy.

### Aberration Versus Ectopy in Atrial Fibrillation

If the atrial rhythm is fibrillation and the presence of atrial premature complexes cannot be used to distinguish intraventricular aberration from ventricular ectopy, the configuration of the premature ventricular complexes becomes the prime criterion for the correct diagnosis. Another helpful feature in differentiating aberration from ectopy is the absence of a fixed coupling interval of the wide QRS complex to the preceding normally conducted complex in the former; fixed coupling suggests ventricular premature beats due to a reentry mechanism. A third feature suggesting intraventricular aberration is the interval between the wide QRS and the following complex: If this is short, intraventricular aberration is likely; whereas if it is long, ectopy is more probable (Fig 14–6). The long interval following a broad QRS complex is due to concealed retrograde conduction of the ventricular impulse into the AV node, resulting in decrement (failure to propagate) of greater numbers of atrial fibrillatory impulses and thus a transient slowing of the ventricular rate. (However, premature ventricular complexes may not be conducted in retrograde fashion; thus, absence of a pause following a premature broad QRS complex does not exclude the diagnosis of ventricular ectopy.)

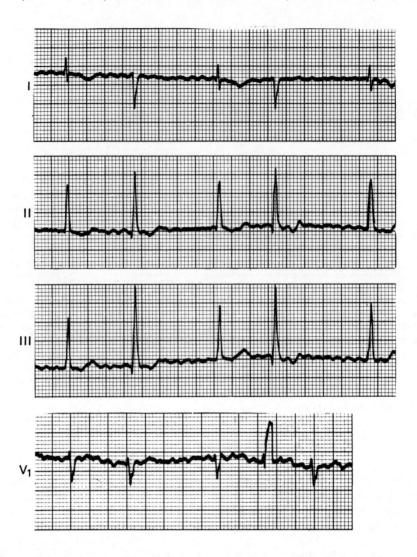

**Figure 14–6.** Atrial fibrillation with premature ventricular complexes versus supraventricular complexes with intraventricular aberration. The second and fourth QRS complexes are wide and have a pattern of left posterior fascicular block, suggesting possible origin in the anterior fascicle of the left bundle branch. There is a long interval between these wide complexes and the subsequent normally conducted complexes, suggesting retrograde conduction of premature ventricular beats into the AV node, delaying antegrade conduction of the fibrillatory impulses. However, the lack of a fixed coupling interval between the normal and aberrant QRS complexes favors intraventricular aberration of supraventricular impulses. Sometimes an intracardiac electrogram is required to arrive at the proper diagnosis.

## TEST TRACINGS

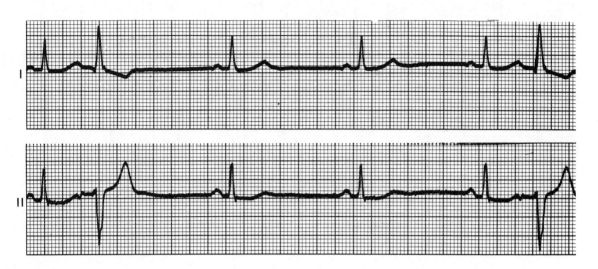

**Figure 14–T1.** Atrial premature complexes with intraventricular aberration. Premature P waves are present in the T waves of the second and sixth QRS complexes. These are followed by wide complexes having a left anterior fascicular block pattern. The presence of the atrial premature complexes indicates that the wide QRS complexes represent intraventricular aberration.

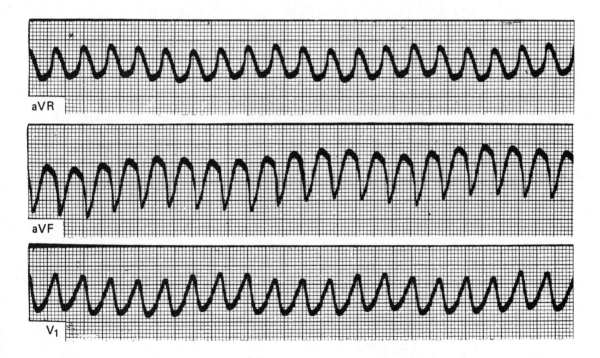

**Figure 14–T2.** A wide complex tachycardia is present at a regular ventricular rate of 200/min. The QRS complexes are broad and bizarre and are directed superiorly (QS in II) and anteriorly (R in $V_1$). There is no definite evidence of atrial activity. Ventricular tachycardia is the most likely diagnosis. However, in view of the absolute regularity of the ventricular complexes, supraventricular tachycardia with aberrant intraventricular conduction must be considered. The tracing shown in Fig 14–3 was recorded just after these rhythm strips were obtained, establishing the diagnosis of supraventricular tachycardia with intraventricular aberration.

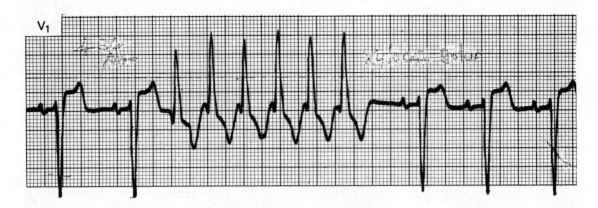

**Figure 14–T3.** Sinus rhythm with a burst of ventricular tachycardia. The burst of wide QRS rhythm is rapid and irregular; it is not preceded by a premature atrial impulse, and the qR morphology of the tachycardia complexes has an opposite initial vector compared to the sinus-conducted QRS complexes in this V₁ rhythm strip. These features indicate that the tachycardia is ventricular in origin.

Continuous recording

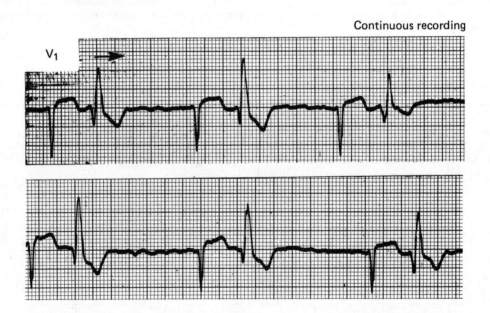

**Figure 14–T4.** Atrial fibrillation with ventricular bigeminy. The QRS complexes stimulated by the fibrillatory impulses have an rS configuration. They are followed at fixed coupling intervals by broad QRS complexes with a qR configuration. Because the initial vector of the premature complexes is opposite in direction to that of the normally conducted complexes, and because the interval between the two is fixed, the premature complexes are ventricular in origin.

# Parasystole | 15

Parasystole is an abnormal rhythm in which 2 pacemakers discharge independently of each other. One pacemaker is the dominant pacemaker of the heart and is therefore usually the sinus node. The parasystolic pacemaker may be located in the atrium (Fig 15–1), the AV junction, or the ventricles (Fig 15–2); ventricular parasystole is the most commonly observed. Iatrogenic parasystolic foci are exemplified by cardiac pacemakers, which compete with spontaneous cardiac rhythm; and by heart transplantations, in which the atrial impulses from both the donor and recipient hearts are visible on the surface ECG. (However, since one of these foci— the recipient's—is incapable of depolarizing ventricular myocardium, this does not represent true parasystole.)

A parasystolic focus generates impulses at about the same rate over long periods of time (up to years); the rates vary between 20/min and 100/min. Parasystolic tachycardia is rare. Parasystolic foci are usually not depolarized by the normal cardiac impulses because of a phenomenon known as **entrance block,** which prevents the normal cardiac depolarization wave front from penetrating the parasystolic foci. And, despite the continuous discharge of impulses by a parasystolic focus, most do not propagate very far outside the focus (**exit block**) and thus do not depolarize the surrounding myocardium. Entrance and exit blocks surrounding a parasystolic focus are usually of high degree, but occasionally first- and second-degree entrance and exit blocks can be demonstrated.

The activation of myocardium from a parasystolic focus will depend upon the state of refractoriness of that myocardium. For example, a ventricular parasystolic complex will be seen on the surface ECG only when the ventricles are nonrefractory and therefore capable of being depolarized. Since the discharge rate of a parasystolic focus is constant— and since some impulses do not exit the focus while others which do cannot depolarize the myocardium because of refractoriness—the complexes that are inscribed have no constant relation to preceding complexes but are multiples of a basic interectopic rate. Not uncommonly, fusion complexes, in which the ventricles (or atria) are stimulated by both the sinus-conducted impulse and the parasystolic impulse, occur. The 3 criteria for the electrocardiographic diagnosis of parasystole are, therefore: (1) absence of a fixed coupling interval between the normally conducted P wave or QRS complex and the parasystolic complex, (2) demonstration of a basic interectopic interval of which the visible parasystolic complexes are multiples, and (3) the occurrence of atrial or ventricular fusion complexes.

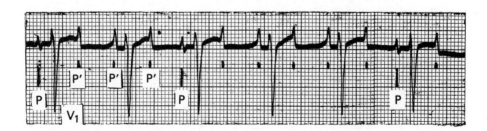

**Figure 15–1.** Atrial parasystole. Sinus P waves occur at a rate of 77/min. Not all sinus P waves (P) are seen, however, because of the presence of a parasystolic tachycardia (P') at 150/min. The AV conduction ratio of the parasystolic rhythm is 2:1.

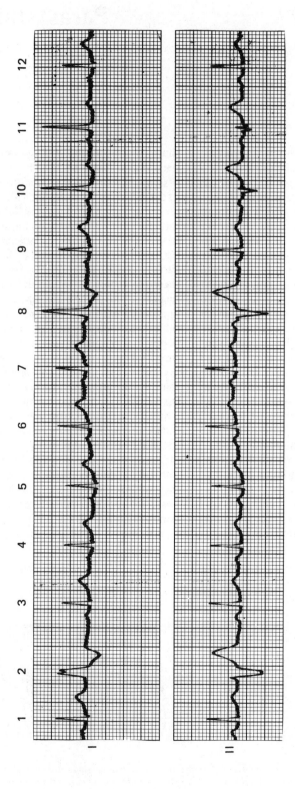

**Figure 15–2.** Ventricular parasystole. Most QRS complexes are sinus-stimulated. The second QRS complex is ventricular in origin and is not preceded by a P wave. The eighth, tenth, and eleventh QRS complexes are preceded by P waves and have configurations intermediate between the sinus-stimulated complexes and the ventricular complex; these are fusion complexes. The intervals between the ventricular and fusion complexes and the preceding normally conducted QRS complexes are not fixed-coupled. The interectopic intervals between the second and eighth complexes = 3.9 s, between the eighth and tenth complexes = 1.3 s, and between the tenth and eleventh complexes = 0.65 s. These intervals are all multiples of 0.65 s, indicating a parasystolic rate of 92/min.

# Preexcitation Syndromes | 16

Ventricular preexcitation is a term used to describe conditions in which ventricular activation occurs earlier than would be expected from activation via the normal AV node-His-Purkinje system. The preexcitation conduction patterns are characterized by specific electrocardiographic features depending upon the particular pathway of ventricular depolarization. The syndromes are associated with a high incidence of tachyarrhythmias. Fig 16–1 illustrates some of the recognized accessory AV conduction pathways. Classification of ventricular preexcitation is as follows (Figs 16–1 and 16–2): (1) AV bypass tracts, which connect atrial tissue directly with the ventricular tissue (Wolff-Parkinson-White [WPW] conduction); (2) nodoventricular fibers, which connect the AV node with the

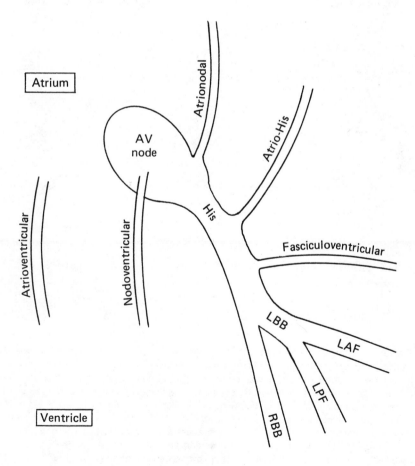

**Figure 16–1.** Schema of accessory pathways. LBB, left bundle branch; LAF, left anterior fascicle; LPF, left posterior fascicle; RBB, right bundle branch.

ventricular myocardium; (3) fasciculoventricular fibers, which connect a fascicle with the ventricular myocardium (Mahaim conduction); (4) AV nodal bypass tracts, which connect atrial fibers with the distal portion of the AV node (James fibers) or His bundle; and (5) intra-AV nodal fibers in which rapid conduction occurs.

## WOLFF-PARKINSON-WHITE CONDUCTION

In WPW conduction, the sinus impulse arises normally in the sinus node. It is then conducted through the atria to the accessory pathway in addition to the normal AV node. The impulse may then be conducted to the ventricles in 3 different ways. First, it can be conducted entirely in the accessory pathway, bypassing the AV node and thus the normally encountered AV nodal conduction delay. This results in a short PR interval (less than 0.10 s). Because AV nodal conduction of the impulse does not occur, the ventricular myocardium is depolarized earlier than normal; this results in the

inscription of a slur at the beginning of the QRS complex—the **delta wave.** Second, the sinus impulse can be conducted entirely in the normal AV node-His-Purkinje system, resulting in a normal PR interval and QRS complex. Third, it can be conducted to the ventricles over both pathways, utilizing each to different degrees depending upon the location of the accessory pathway and the conduction velocities within the pathways; this results in a **fusion complex,** reflecting ventricular depolarization occurring via both the normal AV conduction pathway and the accessory pathway. The PR interval of the fusion complex will be shorter than normal, and the QRS complex may be less or more wide and slurred; the delta wave must be present, however, for the diagnosis of WPW conduction to be made (Fig 16-3).

The electrocardiographic patterns in WPW conduction may mimic myocardial infarction. The delta wave may be oriented superiorly, producing Q waves in II, III, and aVF (Fig 16-4) and simulating inferior wall myocardial infarction; or it may be oriented inferiorly and rightward, producing Q waves in I and aVL, mimicking anterior wall infarc-

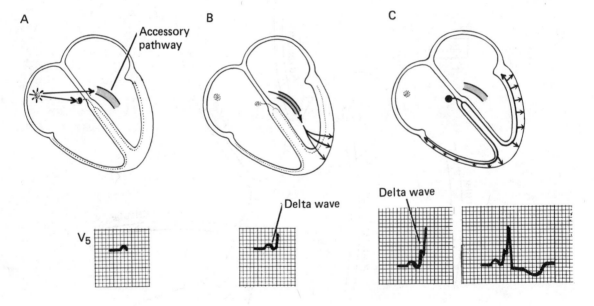

**Figure 16–2.** Diagram of ventricular preexcitation. *A:* The sinus impulse traverses the normal pathways to the AV node and is also conducted to the accessory pathway. *B:* The impulse is conducted rapidly in the accessory AV pathway, directly from atrial to ventricular myocardium, without encountering the normal conduction delay within the AV node (ventricular preexcitation). A **delta wave** is inscribed in the QRS complex, reflecting early activation of the ventricular myocardium. *C:* The impulse is also conducted through the normal AV node-His-Purkinje system to the ventricular myocardium. Because this portion of the impulse does encounter the normal conduction delay in the AV node, it depolarizes a portion of the ventricular myocardium later than that conducted through the accessory pathway. The QRS complex inscribed is therefore a fusion complex, representing ventricular activation occurring via the normal AV node-His-Purkinje system and the accessory AV pathway. Pure normally conducted and pure preexcited complexes may occur; most WPW complexes are fusion complexes. Because ventricular depolarization is abnormal, repolarization is also abnormal, precluding interpretation of ST–T deviations.

A                                B

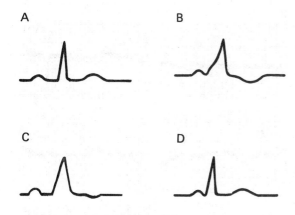

C                                D

**Figure 16–3.** Patterns of ventricular preexcitation. *A:* Normal AV conduction. The P–QRS complex is normal, since the ventricles are depolarized via the normal AV node–His-Purkinje system. *B:* Accessory AV conduction (WPW). The PR interval is short (since the AV node has been bypassed), and the QRS complex has a slur on its upstroke (the delta wave), reflecting early ventricular activation. *C:* Nodoventricular conduction. The PR interval is normal, since the sinus impulse is conducted normally through the AV node. The QRS complex is slurred and exhibits a delta wave, since the ventricular myocardium has been preexcited via the nodoventricular pathway. *D:* Short PR interval with normal QRS complex. The PR interval may be short because of an anatomically short AV node, an intra–AV nodal bypass tract that bypasses the area of normal conduction delay, or a direct atrionodal or atrio-His connection. The QRS complex is normal, since the ventricles are depolarized via the normal His-Purkinje system.

tion. When WPW conduction is present and ventricular depolarization is therefore abnormal, myocardial infarction cannot be read from the ECG.

The electrocardiographic pattern of WPW conduction has no special clinical significance in and of itself; however, patients with this type of ventricular preexcitation are prone to develop paroxysmal reciprocating tachycardias (Fig 16–5) (see Chapter 11), as well as paroxysmal attacks of atrial fibrillation (Fig 16–6). One pathway of reciprocating tachycardia involves normal AV node–His-Purkinje conduction in an antegrade direction and bypass tract conduction in a retrograde direction. The resulting QRS complexes are narrow and normal-appearing, and the tachycardia responds to the usual maneuvers that terminate reentry supraventricular tachycardias. As the bypass tract functions only to conduct impulses in a retrograde direction, it is referred to as a **concealed bypass tract.** The second pathway of reciprocating tachycardia involves bypass tract conduction in an antegrade direction, and AV node-His-Purkinje conduction in a retrograde direction. The resulting QRS complexes will be broad and will have a delta wave,

although the rate of the tachycardia may make the delta wave difficult to discern. This wide complex tachycardia, with its broad and bizarre QRS complexes, may be confused with ventricular tachycardia.

If the patient develops atrial fibrillation and the impulses are conducted in antegrade fashion over the bypass tract, directly from atrial to ventricular myocardium, they do not encounter the normal conduction delay present in the AV node. Because of the direct insertion of the bypass fibers into ventricular tissue, extremely rapid ventricular rates (in excess of 250/min) can occur, resulting in ventricular fibrillation. In contrast, if the patient with atrial fibrillation conducts the fibrillatory impulses down the normal AV node–His-Purkinje system, conduction delay within the AV node will protect the ventricles from such rapid rates.

## NODOVENTRICULAR & FASCICULOVENTRICULAR CONDUCTION

Nodoventricular and fasciculoventricular connections are relatively uncommon. They are recognized by a normal PR interval (since the atrial impulses pass through the AV node and encounter the normal delay in AV conduction) and a wide QRS complex with a delta wave (since the ventricles are preexcited via the nodoventricular fibers) (Figs 16–1 and 16–7). Like WPW conduction, the PR interval and the QRS complex configuration will reflect the degree to which the ventricles are depolarized via the normal and accessory pathways.

## SHORT PR INTERVAL & NORMAL QRS COMPLEX

The electrocardiographic pattern of a short PR interval and a normal QRS configuration could be due to an anatomically short AV node, an intra–AV nodal bypass tract with rapid conduction, or a direct connection between atrial fibers and the distal portion of the AV node (atrionodal connection) or His bundle (atrio-His connection) (Fig 16–1). Since ventricular depolarization occurs over the normal His-Purkinje pathway, the QRS complexes are normal (Fig 16–8).

Most patients with a short PR interval and a normal QRS complex have an intra–AV nodal bypass tract. Impulse conduction in this tract is very rapid and, because of preferential conduction of supraventricular impulses in this pathway, the normal conduction delay encountered in other portions of the AV node does not occur.

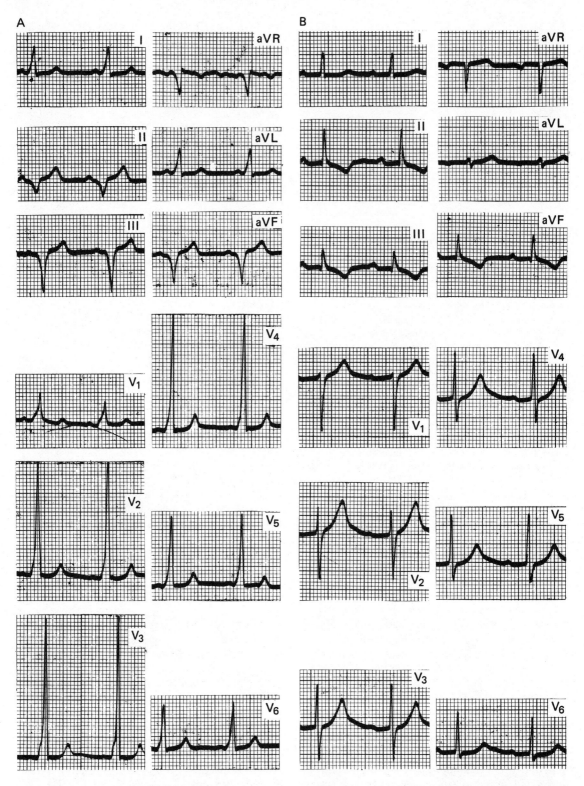

**Figure 16–4.** Ventricular preexcitation (WPW conduction) (A) reverting to normal (B). *A:* WPW conduction. The PR interval = 0.10 s. A positive delta wave is present in I, aVL, and V₄₋₅, and a negative delta wave is seen in II, III, and aVF. The negative delta wave should not be confused with the Q wave of myocardial infarction. *B:* After treatment with quinidine, which has caused conduction delay in the accessory AV pathway to exceed that in the AV node, conduction of the sinus impulses is occurring normally via the AV node–His-Purkinje system. The PR interval is normal, and the QRS complexes do not show delta waves.

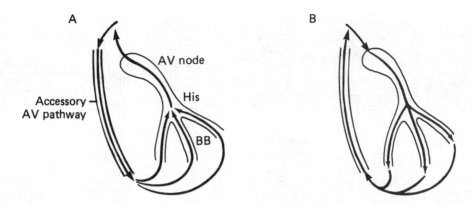

**Figure 16–5.** Diagrams of mechanisms of reciprocating supraventricular tachycardias in accessory AV conduction (WPW). *A:* Antegrade conduction over the accessory AV pathway and retrograde conduction through the bundle branches (BB), bundle of His, and AV node. The QRS complexes will show the preexcitation pattern. *B:* Antegrade conduction down the normal AV node–His-Purkinje system and retrograde conduction in the accessory pathway. The QRS complexes will appear normal. Retrograde conduction in an accessory pathway is *concealed,* since it is not visible on the surface ECG. The pathway itself is termed a **concealed bypass tract.** If the ventricles are depolarized via the accessory AV pathway and the patient develops rapid atrial arrhythmias such as flutter or fibrillation, the ventricular rate can be extremely rapid, leading to ventricular fibrillation.

The electrocardiographic pattern of a short PR interval and a normal QRS complex is itself of no significance. However, patients with intra-AV nodal bypass tracts are prone to develop reciprocating tachycardias that involve reentry within the AV node (Lown-Ganong-Levine syndrome). The QRS complexes during tachycardia in these patients are narrow and normal-appearing, in contrast to those involving an AV bypass tract.

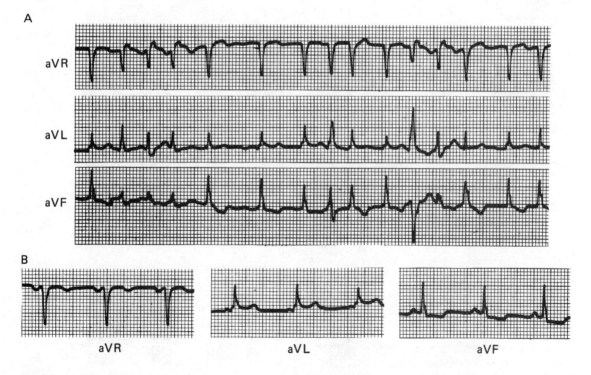

**Figure 16–6.** *A:* Atrial fibrillation in a patient with WPW syndrome. The QRS complexes reflect varying degrees of fusion. The ventricular rate is at times extremely rapid, approaching 240/min. Rapid ventricular rates reflect the direct transmission of atrial fibrillatory impulses into ventricular tissue via the AV bypass tract. *B:* After DC cardioversion, sinus rhythm is restored. The PR interval = 0.08 s, and a delta wave is seen in aVL.

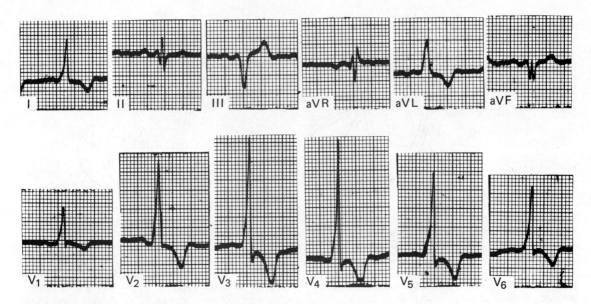

**Figure 16–7.** Nodoventricular conduction. A delta wave is seen in I, aVL, and all precordial leads; it is negative in II and aVF and should not be confused with the Q wave of myocardial infarction. Since the PR interval is normal at 0.14 s, the sinus impulse has been conducted through the AV node, after which it preexcites the ventricles.

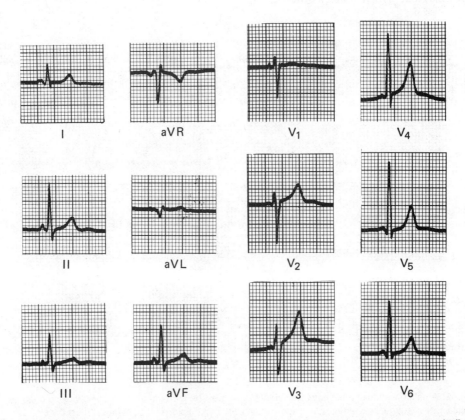

**Figure 16–8.** Short PR interval due to intra–AV nodal, atrionodal, or atrio-His bypass tracts or to an anatomically short AV node. Since the ventricles are depolarized via the normal His-Purkinje system, the QRS complexes are normal.

## TEST TRACINGS

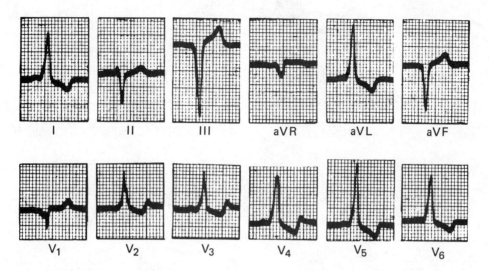

**Figure 16–T1.** Ventricular preexcitation due to AV bypass tract (WPW conduction). The atrial rhythm is sinus, the PR interval = 0.10 s, and the QRS duration = 0.12 s. There is leftward axis deviation. Delta waves are seen in I, aVL, and $V_{2-6}$. Because ventricular depolarization is abnormal (occurring over an accessory AV pathway), repolarization is abnormal, and interpretation of the ST segments and T waves is not possible. Similarly, voltage criteria for ventricular hypertrophy cannot be applied, and myocardial infarction cannot be diagnosed.

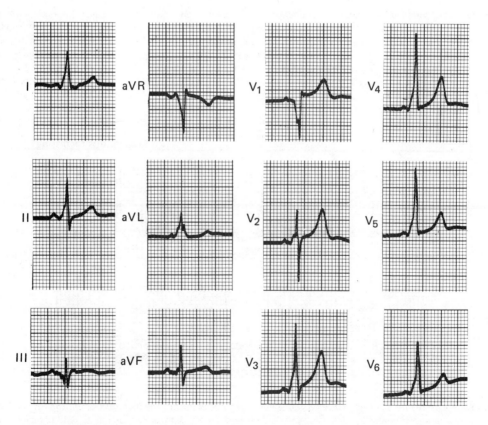

**Figure 16–T2.** Preexcitation (WPW conduction). The PR interval = 0.10 s. The QRS complexes are wide, and a delta wave is seen in I, II, aVL, aVF, and $V_{2-6}$. The delta wave is negative in III, aVR, and $V_1$ and should not be confused with a Q wave of myocardial infarction.

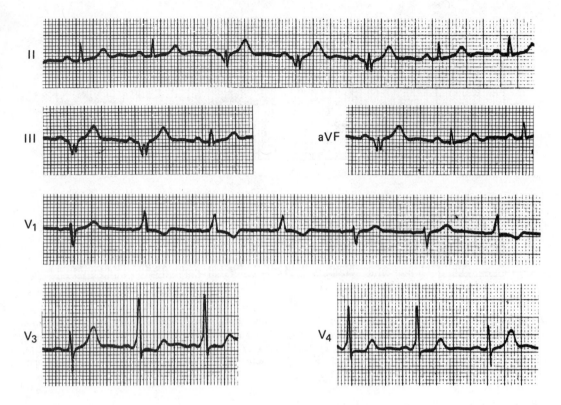

**Figure 16–T3.** Pseudoinfarction pattern in a patient with WPW conduction. The rhythm is sinus. Interspersed between normal-appearing QRS complexes are abnormal complexes with deep, wide Q waves in leads II, III, and aVF and large R waves in $V_1$. The PR interval of the normal complexes = 0.18 s. The abnormal complexes have a PR interval of 0.12 s, and a delta wave is seen in $V_3$ and $V_4$. This represents intermittent ventricular preexcitation. The pseudo–Q waves in the inferior leads are negative delta waves. Such a tracing (in the absence of the normal QRS complexes) could be interpreted as showing inferior and posterior myocardial infarction or inferior infarction with a right ventricular conduction defect. (Courtesy of S Edwards.)

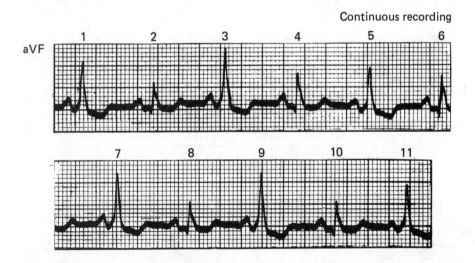

**Figure 16–T4.** Accessory AV conduction (WPW) with varying degrees of fusion. The rhythm is sinus. The PR intervals vary according to the pattern of ventricular depolarization. The second, fourth, sixth, eighth, and tenth QRS complexes have a normal PR interval and a qR configuration; no delta wave is present. The alternate QRS complexes have a shorter PR interval and exhibit a delta wave (which obscures the normal pattern of ventricular depolarization). This tracing represents 2:1 conduction in the accessory AV pathway.

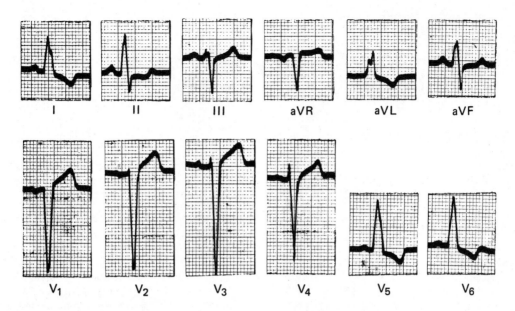

**Figure 16–T5.** Left bundle branch block. The rhythm is sinus, the PR interval = 0.12 s, the QRS duration = 0.12 s, and the mean frontal plane QRS axis = 0 degrees. There are wide, notched R waves in leads I, aVL, and $V_{5-6}$, and the ventricular activation time in aVL = 0.1 s. The ST segments are depressed and the T waves inverted in these leads. The normal PR interval and absence of a true slur (delta wave) on the upstroke of the QRS complexes exclude the diagnosis of accessory AV (WPW) conduction.

# 17 | Effect of Drugs & Electrolytes on the Electrocardiogram

## DIGITALIS

### Digitalis Effect

Digitalis administration commonly produces ST segment depression in ventricular epicardial leads. The characteristic ST segment changes are a "scooped" ST configuration or an oblique line descending from the J point (Figs 17–1 and 17–2). Because of the ST segment depression, the T wave may be dragged downward, resembling T wave inversion. As a result of a shortening of electrical systole in digitalized patients, the QT interval shortens, but this is not usually measurable from the routine ECG.

PR interval prolongation (first-degree AV block) is a common finding in digitalized patients; some consider it a sign of digitalis toxicity. Measurement of the serum digitalis levels may be helpful in assessing whether or not the PR interval prolongation is due to digitalis effect or toxicity.

### Digitalis Toxicity (Figs 17–3 through 17–7)

While any arrhythmia may result from digitalis intoxication, the most commonly encountered ones are listed in Table 17–1. Sinus bradycardia due to sinus arrest or SA exit block may occur in patients with high vagal tone or those in whom sympathetic tone is diminished. Atrial flutter and fibrillation are uncommon manifestations of digitalis toxicity. When the underlying atrial rhythm is fibrillation, the diagnosis of digitalis toxicity can be made from the recognition of high-degree AV block, with a regular QRS rhythm originating in junctional or ventricular tissue. Exit block from the focus of origin of the QRS rhythm is also seen. Ventricular ectopic impulses may occur. Table 17–2 lists the manifestations of digitalis intoxication in patients with atrial fibrillation.

## TYPE I ANTIARRHYTHMIC DRUGS (Quinidine, Procainamide, & Disopyramide)

While all type I antiarrhythmic agents are capable of producing similar electrocardiographic abnormalities, quinidine is the drug most commonly implicated. Quinidine can produce ST segment depression and flattening and inversion of the T waves in left ventricular epicardial leads, in a fashion similar to digitalis (Fig 17–8). However, prolongation of the QTU interval because of the

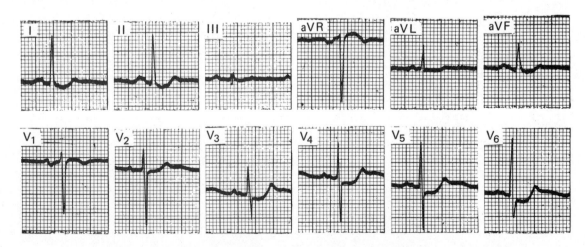

**Figure 17–1.** Digitalis effect. Scooped ST segment depression is present in I, II, aVF, and V$_{2-6}$.

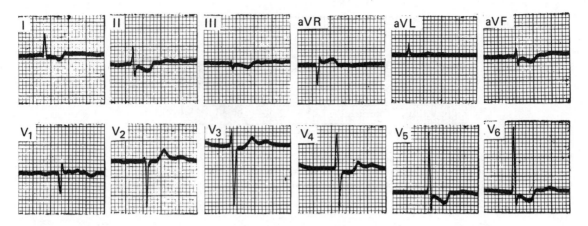

**Figure 17–2.** Digitalis effect. The rhythm is atrial fibrillation. The ST segment depression produces an oblique downward ST segment in leads I, II, III, aVF, and $V_{5-6}$. The T waves are dragged downward. Prominent U waves are best seen in $V_{2-4}$; U waves are not indicative of digitalis effect, although digitalis may enhance their amplitude.

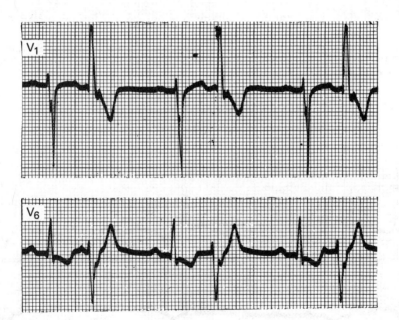

**Figure 17–3.** Sinus rhythm with ventricular bigeminy due to digitalis toxicity. Ventricular premature complexes follow each sinus-conducted QRS at a fixed coupling interval. ST segment depression and T wave inversion in the sinus-conducted beats is seen in $V_6$; however, since each sinus-conducted beat is a postextrasystolic one, correct interpretation of ST–T abnormalities is often difficult. The sinus rate is not measurable when ventricular bigeminy is present. Although ventricular bigeminy in this patient was associated with a toxic serum level of digoxin, this arrhythmia is not specific for digitalis intoxication.

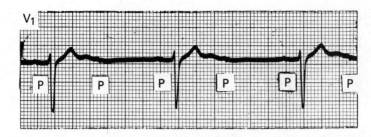

**Figure 17–4.** Second-degree AV block due to digitalis toxicity. The AV conduction ratio is 2:1, the sinus rate is 86/min, and the ventricular rate is 43/min. The PR interval of the conducted P waves is within normal limits. The QRS complexes are narrow. Since bundle branch block is not present, the conduction block is probably occurring within the AV node.

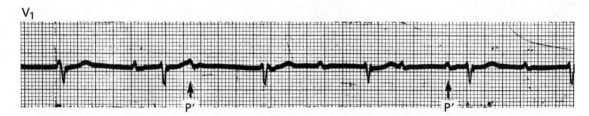

**Figure 17–5.** Complete AV block due to digitalis toxicity. The atrial rate is 66/min (nonconducted atrial premature beats [P′] are also present) and the ventricular rate is 52/min. The QRS complexes are narrow, suggesting that the focus of origin of the QRS rhythm is in the AV junction or His bundle.

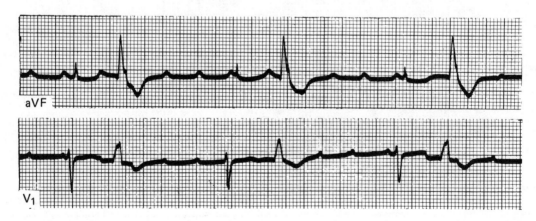

**Figure 17–6.** Atrial tachycardia with AV block and ventricular bigeminy, resulting from digitalis toxicity. The atrial rate is 164/min and independent of the QRS rhythm. The QRS complexes are narrow, suggesting an AV junctional origin. Following each narrow QRS complex, a ventricular premature complex occurs (ventricular bigeminy). Because the intervals between the premature ventricular complexes and the normal-appearing complexes are regular, and because the premature complexes occur at fixed coupling intervals to the normal complexes, the QRS rhythm is presumed to be regular.

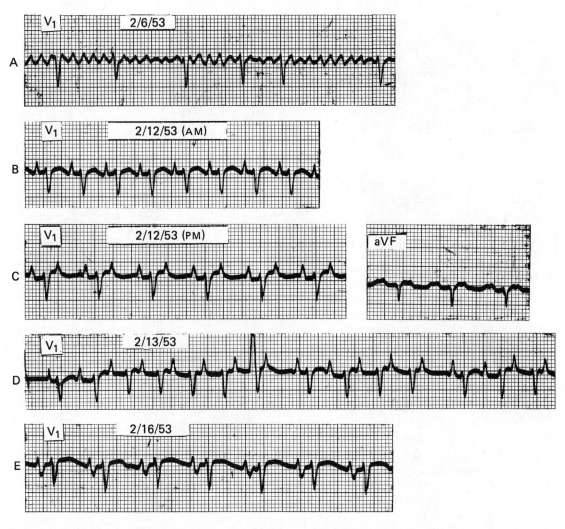

**Figure 17–7.** Digitalis toxicity resulting in atrial tachycardia with AV block. *A:* Atrial fibrillation with irregular ventricular rate is present. *B:* Atrial tachycardia at a rate of 160/min with 1:1 AV conduction is now present. The sudden appearance of atrial tachycardia during treatment of atrial fibrillation with digitalis should raise the suspicion of digitalis intoxication. *C:* After additional digitalis, AV block has occurred, resulting in an atrial tachycardia with 2:1 AV conduction; an increase in the atrial rate has also occurred. *D:* Atrial tachycardia remains when the digitalis is discontinued, but the 2:1 AV block has been replaced by type I (Wenckebach) second-degree AV block, and more 1:1 AV conduction of atrial impulses is present. *E:* Resumption of sinus rhythm.

**Table 17–1.** Electrocardiographic manifestations of digitalis toxicity (Figs 17–3 through 17–7).

Automatic or triggered arrhythmias
  Ventricular premature complexes
    Bigeminy, trigeminy
    R-on-T premature complexes
    Multiform complexes
  Ventricular tachycardia
  Ventricular fibrillation
  Atrial tachycardia (often with AV block)
  Accelerated junctional rhythm (with AV dissociation)
  Junctional tachycardia (with AV dissociation)
AV block
  Second-degree, type I (Wenckebach)
  High-degree or complete

**Table 17–2.** Electrocardiographic manifestations of digitalis toxicity in the presence of atrial fibrillation.

Regular QRS rhythm (reflecting subsidiary pacemaker with origin in the AV junction, bundle branches, or distal Purkinje tissue)
QRS rhythm with episodic type II (2:1, 3:1) exit block (occurring in any portion of the AV node–His-Purkinje system)
QRS rhythm with periodicity suggesting type I (Wenckebach) exit block (occurring in any portion of the AV node–His-Purkinje system)
Ventricular arrhythmias

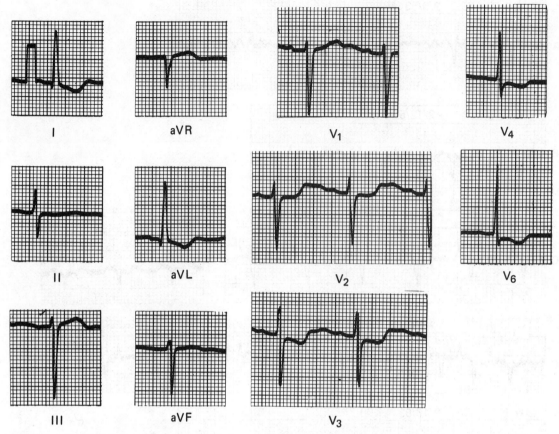

**Figure 17–8.** Quinidine effect. The rhythm is sinus; the PR interval = 0.20 s. The pattern of left ventricular hypertrophy with associated ST–T wave changes is present. The ST–T abnormalities in $V_{2-3}$ may be contributed to by quinidine. The QTU interval is prolonged to 0.60 s and represents an effect of quinidine. Since the QTU interval does not correlate directly with the serum level of the drug, prolongation of this interval does not predict the presence of quinidine toxicity.

development of a prominent U wave is the most commonly observed electrocardiographic change.

Toxic electrocardiographic manifestations of quinidine therapy (as well as all type I antiarrhythmic agents in certain patients) are as follows: (1) prolongation of the QRS duration, reflecting the effect of quinidine on the conduction velocity in the bundle branches-Purkinje system; (2) ventricular arrhythmias, including ventricular tachycardia (often polymorphic) and fibrillation; (3) ventricular standstill; (4) sinus bradycardia due to SA exit block or slowing of impulse formation (or both); (5) atrial standstill; (6) first-, second-, and third-degree AV block; and (7) AV dissociation. The toxic manifestations of quinidine are an extension of its therapeutic effects of slowing the rate of discharge of an ectopic focus and producing local conduction block.

A particular type of ventricular tachycardia, termed **torsade de pointes,** can occur in patients receiving type I antiarrhythmic agents. This is a polymorphic, irregular, usually nonsustained ventricular tachycardia, in which the QRS complexes appear to twist about an isoelectric baseline (Fig 17–9). While not entirely specific for type I antiarrhythmic therapy (this tachycardia has been seen during amiodarone treatment and as a result of a long QT interval due to hypokalemia or congenital QT prolongation), its occurrence is a contraindication to the further use of these medications.

## PHENOTHIAZINES & RELATED DRUGS

The phenothiazines and the antidepressant agents imipramine, amitriptyline, and related compounds are myocardial depressants that impair AV and intraventricular conduction (Fig 17–10). With excessive doses, ST segment depression, T wave flattening and inversion, and prolongation of the QT interval with prominent U waves occur. Eventually, both AV and intraventricular conduction disturbances arise, similar to type I antiarrhythmic drug toxicity.

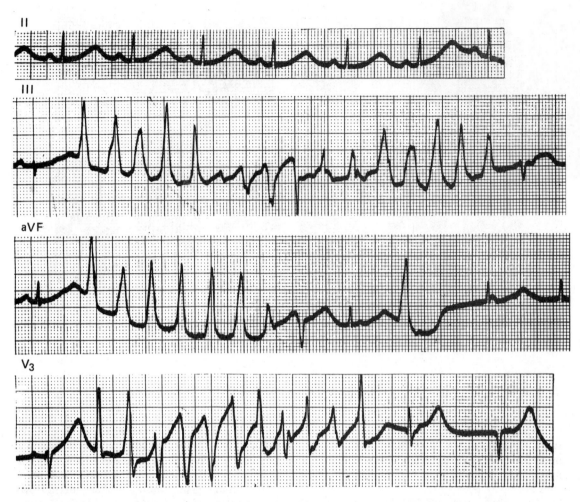

**Figure 17–9.** Polymorphic ventricular tachycardia **(torsade de pointes)** due to quinidine toxicity. The QRS configurations change from upright to inverted in any given lead during the tachycardia. The tachycardia occurs in bursts and terminates spontaneously. Note the markedly prolonged QT interval, which results in the first beat of the tachycardia constituting an R-on-T premature ventricular complex.

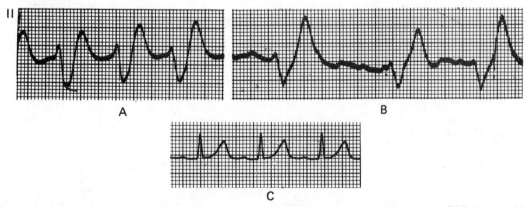

**Figure 17–10.** Amitriptyline toxicity due to an overdose in a suicide attempt. **A:** A wide complex QRS rhythm without discernible atrial activity is present. This could represent sinus rhythm with sinoventricular conduction (due to atrial arrest), junctional rhythm with intraventricular aberration, or ventricular rhythm. **B:** With supportive treatment, the atrial rhythm is now fibrillation. The QRS rhythm is irregular and is thus responding to the fibrillatory impulses. The QRS complexes are less broad and bizarre than in (A). **C:** Normal sinus rhythm restored, with prolongation of the QT interval to 0.46 s. The QRS configuration is normal.

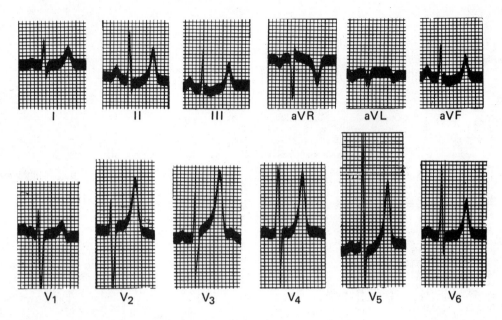

**Figure 17–11.** Hyperkalemia. Tall, slender, tented T waves are seen in I, II, III, aVF, and $V_{2-6}$. The T wave amplitude is a much less specific criterion for hyperkalemia than is its peaked configuration.

## HYPERKALEMIA

Although a reasonably good correlation between serum potassium level and the ECG exists, the ECG actually reflects the *gradient* between myocardial intracellular and extracellular potassium ions.

The initial electrocardiographic evidence of elevated extracellular potassium level is the appearance of slender, narrow-based, "tented" T waves, often best seen in the precordial leads. The peaked T waves are often, but not always, tall. Therefore, although tall T waves might suggest hyperkalemia, they are by no means diagnostic of it, since normal individuals and patients with posterior wall myocardial infarction may show a similar pattern. However, *peaking* of the T waves should raise a suspicion of hyperkalemia (Figs 17–11 through 17–13).

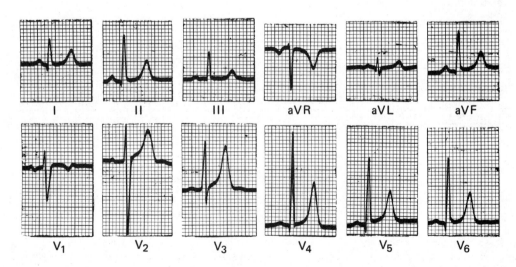

**Figure 17–12.** Normal ECG which might suggest hyperkalemia. The T waves in leads I, II, aVF, and $V_{2-6}$ are tall and somewhat peaked, but they do not have a narrow base and thus are not "tented." Tall T waves do not themselves indicate hyperkalemia.

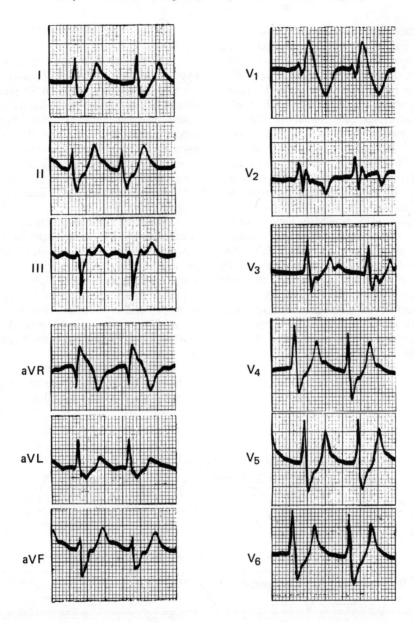

**Figure 17–13.** Hyperkalemia (serum potassium = 8.9 meq/L). The rhythm is sinus. The PR interval is prolonged, but the exact PR interval cannot be determined, however, because the P waves interrupt the T waves of the preceding QRS complexes. The QRS complexes are broad (0.16 s) and have a right bundle branch block pattern. Tented, peaked T waves are present in the lateral precordial leads.

With further elevation of serum potassium, the P waves disappear, and the QRS complexes become broad and bizarre in configuration (Fig 17–13). While the QRS rhythm might suggest a ventricular focus of origin, intracardiac electrographic studies indicate that it might arise from the bundle of His, with marked intraventricular conduction delay, or from the sinus node. The latter rhythm is termed **sinoventricular conduction** and represents sinus rhythm, with the sinus impulses being transmitted via intra-atrial conduction tissue to the AV node and thence to the ventricles. Despite transmission of the sinus impulse through the atria, the atrial muscle fails to be depolarized because of the hyperkalemia. Because atrial depolarization does not occur, P waves are not inscribed on the surface ECG. The diagnosis is confirmed when, upon treatment of the hyperkalemia, P waves appear that have the same rate as the prior QRS rhythm (Fig 11–8).

ST segment elevation is occasionally seen with severe hyperkalemia (Fig 17–14), possibly representing local hyperkalemia associated with myocardial necrosis.

## HYPOKALEMIA

The typical electrocardiographic features of hypokalemia are inscription of a prominent U wave, PR interval prolongation, and ST segment depression in left ventricular epicardial leads. The prominent U wave is due to prolonged Purkinje system repolarization; the U wave is often superimposed upon the T wave of the preceding QRS complex and is not always readily distinguished from it. Thus, a long "QT" interval may in fact represent a long QTU interval, the actual QT interval being normal (Fig 17–15).

Prominent U waves are not diagnostic of hypokalemia, as they also occur in the course of therapy with type I antiarrhythmic drugs, amiodarone, phenothiazines, or tricyclic antidepressants, and in the hereditary long QT interval syndromes. U waves may also be seen in left ventricular hypertrophy and in acute and chronic ischemic heart disease. However, a **giant U wave** that exceeds the T wave in amplitude is strongly suggestive of electrolyte imbalance.

A **postextrasystolic U wave** is a term applied to the appearance of a prominent U wave in a postextrasystolic P–QRST complex, where it was not

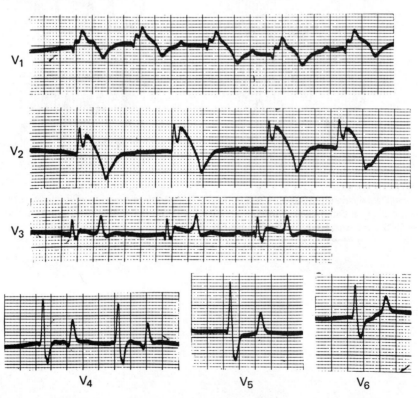

**Figure 17–14.** ST segment elevation, especially noteworthy in leads V$_{1–2}$, due to hyperkalemia (serum potassium = 9.3 meq/L). Tented T waves are seen in V$_{3–6}$. Note that they are peaked, although not tall. Tall T waves are not diagnostic of hyperkalemia, whereas tented T waves strongly suggest this diagnosis.

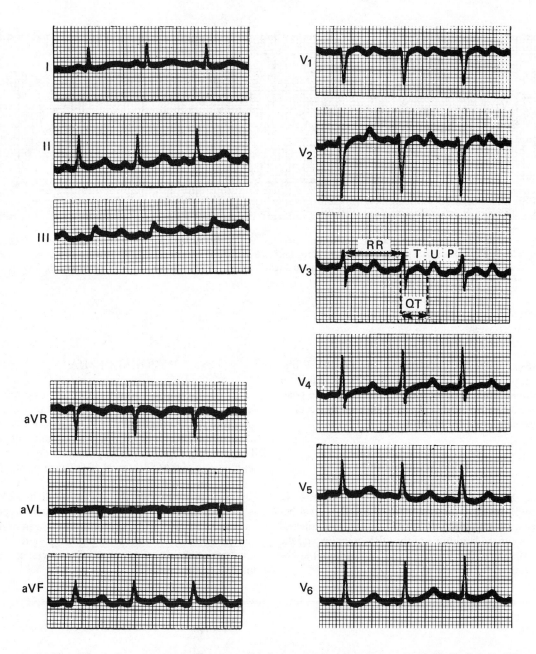

**Figure 17–15.** Hypokalemia (serum potassium = 2.3 meq/L). An apparently upright T wave is seen in leads II, III, aVF, and V$_{5-6}$. If this deflection were the T wave, the QT interval would be 0.40 s (corrected for the RR interval of 0.66 s, the QT$_C$ = 0.50 s) and therefore prolonged. In leads V$_{1-4}$ separate T and U waves are clearly evident. The true QT interval in V$_3$ is 0.29 s (QT$_C$ = 0.36 s), which is normal. Whereas a prominent U wave has many causes, a **giant U wave,** which exceeds the height of the T wave in the same lead, should raise the suspicion of hypokalemia.

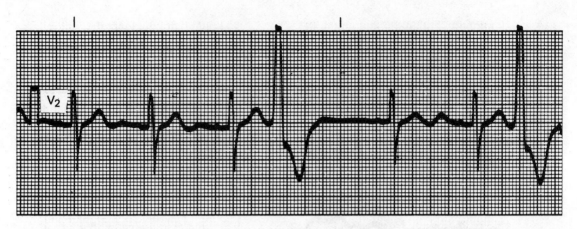

**Figure 17–16.** Postextrasystolic U wave. The rhythm is sinus. U waves can be seen throughout the rhythm strip; however, the U wave of the sinus beat following the premature ventricular complex is markedly accentuated in amplitude. Although the diagnosis of hypokalemia should be considered, postextrasystolic U wave accentuation is a nonspecific finding.

present in the basic complexes (Fig 17–16). While this phenomenon might suggest the diagnosis of hypokalemia, it is not specific for it, because postextrasystolic T and U wave changes may occur in various clinical conditions.

## HYPERCALCEMIA

Elevation of serum calcium levels to above 12 mg/dL results in shortening of the QT interval because of shortening of the QT segment (the interval between the beginning of the QRS complex and the beginning of the T wave). The QT segment may be obliterated in severe hypercalcemia.

## HYPOCALCEMIA

Low levels of serum calcium produce a lengthening of the QT interval that is due to prolongation of the QT segment (the interval between the onset of the QRS complex and the beginning of the T wave) (Fig 17–17). It is important to distinguish lengthening of the QT interval due to inscription of a U wave from that due to prolongation of the QT segment. In the former, the electrolyte disturbance is hypokalemia, whereas in the latter it is hypocalcemia. Occasionally, hypomagnesemia may result in a similar electrocardiographic pattern, but this rarely occurs as the sole electrolyte abnormality.

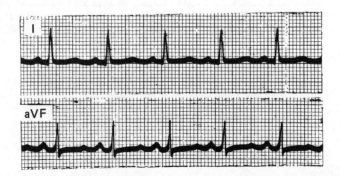

**Figure 17–17.** Hypocalcemia (serum calcium = 6.8 mg/dL). The QT interval is prolonged to 0.40 s ($QT_c$ = 0.48 s). The lengthening of the QT interval is due to a prolongation of the QT segment and not to any abnormality of the T wave itself.

# TEST TRACINGS

Continuous recording

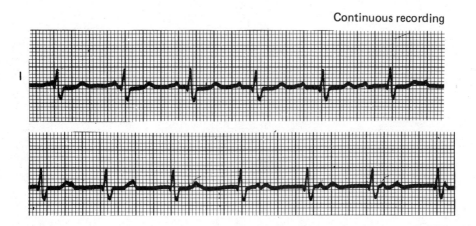

**Figure 17–T1.** Sinus rhythm and junctional rhythm with AV dissociation, due to digitalis toxicity. The atrial rate is 83/min; the ventricular rate is 80/min. The P waves are independent of the QRS complexes and thus dissociated from them. Capture, the hallmark of AV dissociation and the phenomenon excluding the presence of complete AV block, in which an *early* QRS complex is preceded by the P wave that stimulates it, often requires the recording of long rhythm strips. In this case, the AV dissociation resulted from an **accelerated junctional rhythm** due to digitalis toxicity.

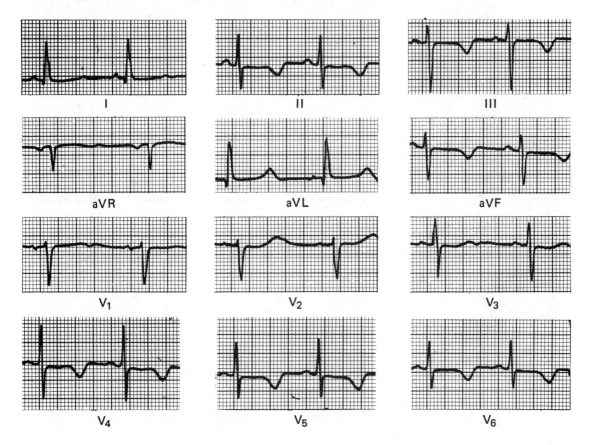

**Figure 17–T2.** Hereditary prolongation of the QT interval. In addition to a prominent U wave (best seen in $V_3$), the QT interval itself is prolonged to 0.58 s. The clinical diagnosis cannot be made from the ECG alone, as this pattern may be seen in hypokalemia and in type I antiarrhythmic drug therapy. However, in the latter circumstances, the QT interval itself is usually normal, and a prominent (often giant) U wave prolongs the *QTU* interval. Not infrequently, the U wave will blend with the T wave, resulting in the inability to distinguish the two (as exemplified in all leads in this tracing except $V_{2-3}$).

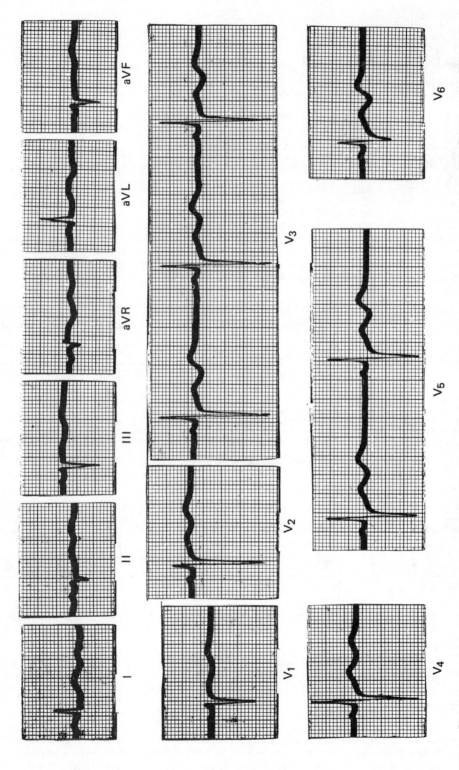

**Figure 17–T3.** Digitalis and quinidine therapy, with hypokalemia. The rhythm is sinus bradycardia. A markedly prolonged QTU interval of 0.51 s is present, which, corrected for the sinus rate of 37/min, is 0.39 s; the QT interval itself is normal. The giant U waves in V$_{2-3}$ suggest hypokalemia or type I antiarrhythmic drug therapy. The ST depression in lead I represents digitalis effect. The serum potassium in this patient was 2.5 meq/L. While the presence of U waves is not itself diagnostic of hypokalemia, giant U waves should suggest this condition.

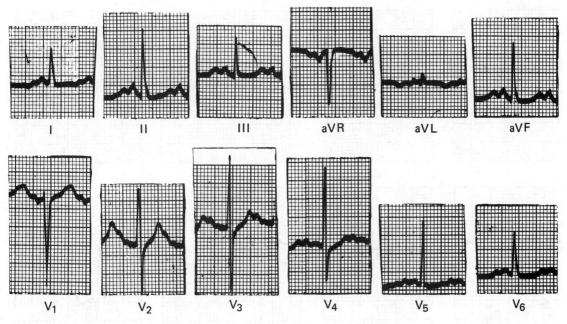

**Figure 17–T4.** Hypokalemia (serum potassium = 2.6 meq/L). The precordial leads show a normal QT interval, with a superimposed U wave that cannot be distinguished from the T wave in the limb leads.

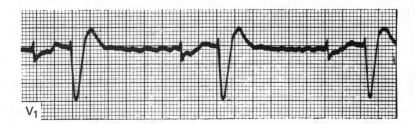

**Figure 17–T5.** Atrial fibrillation, ventricular bigeminy, and regularization of ventricular rate due to digitalis toxicity. The coupling intervals between the narrow QRS complexes and the ventricular premature complexes are fixed. The intervals between the premature ventricular complexes and the following narrow QRS complexes is also fixed, suggesting regularization of the ventricular rhythm. This indicates high-degree AV block of the fibrillatory impulses and origin of the narrow QRS rhythm in the AV junction. Because of the ventricular bigeminy, the true ventricular rate cannot be determined.

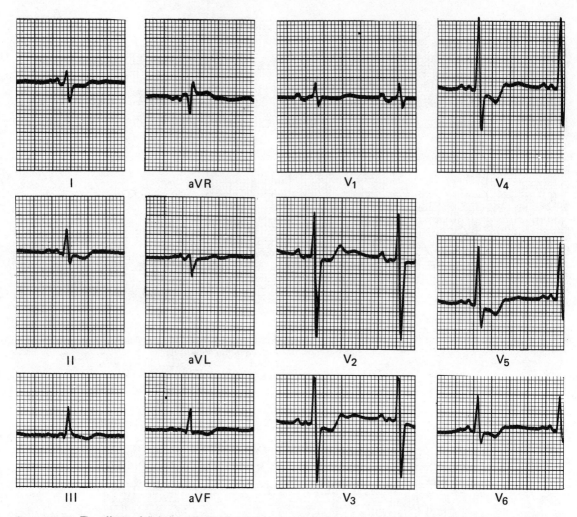

**Figure 17–T6.** The effects of digitalis and quinidine therapy in a patient with mitral stenosis. The rhythm is sinus. The mean frontal plane QRS axis is +105 degrees, the R wave exceeds the S wave in $V_1$, and the P waves suggest left atrial abnormality. These findings are consistent with the clinical diagnosis of mitral stenosis. There is diffuse ST segment depression, consistent with digitalis therapy. The QT interval is normal, but a prominent U wave and a long QTU interval are present, compatible with quinidine treatment.

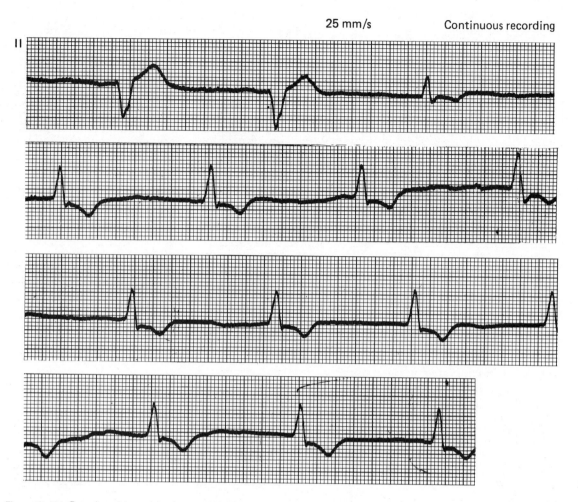

25 mm/s Continuous recording

**Figure 17–T7.** Procainamide toxicity in a patient with renal failure and normal serum electrolytes. Atrial activity is not discernible. The ventricular rhythm is irregular at an average rate of about 37/min. The QRS complexes are broad and bizarre and of 3 different configurations: rS, Rs (third QRS complex, which may represent a fusion complex), and pure R. The prolonged duration of the QRS complexes and their slow rate suggest a focus of origin in ventricular tissue, but in the presence of procainamide toxicity this is not certain.

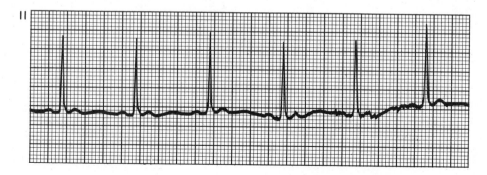

**Figure 17–T8.** Hypercalcemia (serum calcium = 21 mg/dL). The rhythm is sinus, and the PR interval is normal. The QT interval is extremely short at 0.25 s due to the virtual absence of the QT segment.

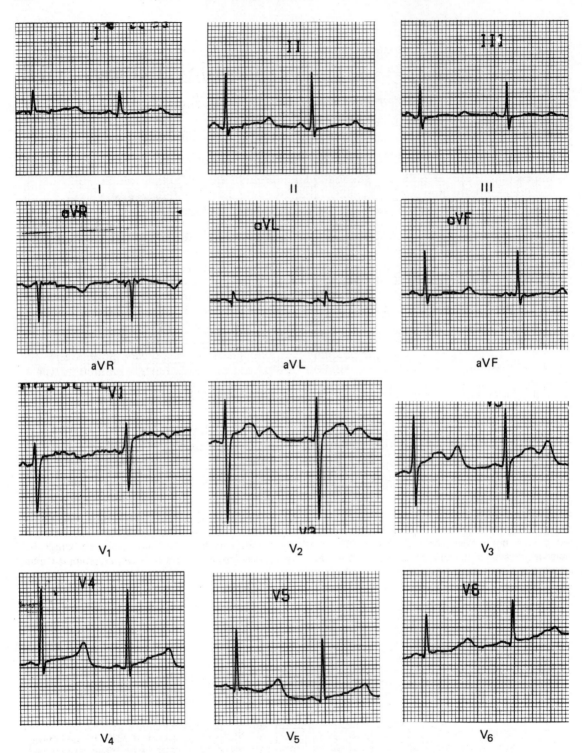

**Figure 17–T9.** Long QTU interval with giant U wave, due to procainamide therapy. The serum potassium was normal. The apparent QT interval as measured in the limb leads is 0.60 s and at first inspection appears to be due to prolongation of the QT segment, suggesting hypocalcemia. However, the precordial leads display large U waves that exceed the amplitude of the T wave in leads $V_{3-6}$. The QT segment is of normal duration. The QT interval, measured from leads $V_{2-3}$, = 0.40 s, and the QTU interval = 0.60 s. This ECG illustrates the value of recording simultaneous leads in identifying the true QRST configuration.

Temporary or permanent cardiac pacing, in which an electrical stimulus results in depolarization of cardiac tissue, is indicated in any situation in which bradycardia results in symptoms of cerebral hypoperfusion or hemodynamic decompensation. Temporary cardiac pacing is accomplished by transvenous insertion of electrodes into the right atrium or right ventricle (or both). Permanent pacing is effected by the same transvenous route and, in some circumstances, by epicardial placement of electrodes via thoracotomy or a subxiphoid approach. Most pacing systems today are placed transvenously.

### Pacemaker Identification Code

Because of the complexity of pacing system design, an identification code describing the function of the available pacemaker generators has been developed. The code consists of 5 letters. The first letter stands for the chamber paced (atrium [A], ventricle [V], or both or double [D]). The second letter stands for the chamber in which sensing the electrical signal occurs (atrium [A], ventricle [V], both [D], or neither [O]). The third letter refers to the mode of response of the generator to a sensed signal (inhibited output [I], triggered output [T] in which an output pulse is delivered upon sensing an electrical signal, and not applicable [0]). The fourth letter stands for the type of changes that can be made noninvasively and reversibly in several pacemaker generators, called **programmability** (rate or energy output only [or both] [S], or multiple functions including rate, energy output, ability to sense an electrical signal of varying magnitude, refractory period after a sensed or paced beat, and other more complex variables [M]). The fifth letter stands for the response of the pulse generator to sensing tachycardias and reflects the antitachycardia function available in some pacemaker generators.

## TYPES OF CARDIAC PACING

### Asynchronous Pacing (VOO, AOO, & DOO)

Asynchronous pacemakers do not sense any electrical signals. Thus, they deliver output pulses without regard to any spontaneous electrical activity occurring within the heart. Because spontaneous cardiac activity is not sensed, competitive rhythms may result. Whereas asynchronous pacemaker generators were the first devices available and are no longer manufactured, asynchronous pacing occurs whenever a magnet is placed over an implanted generator in order to evaluate pacing function. With a magnet in place, asynchronous pacing and concomitant occurrence of the patient's spontaneous rhythm result in iatrogenic parasystole (Fig 18–1). At the energy output of today's generators, repetitive ventricular or atrial rhythms are usually not observed, although this possibility exists.

### Demand Pacing (VVI, AAI, VVT, & AAT)

Both sensing and pacing circuits are present in these units. Upon sensing a spontaneous intracardiac signal, some generators (VVI and AAI) will have inhibition of their output pulses, and no pacemaker artifact will appear (Fig 18–2). Other generators are designed to deliver an output pulse when an electrical event is sensed; this is termed a **triggered response** (VVT and AAT). The triggered output pulse falls within the sensed complex and does not contribute to activation of the cardiac chamber (Fig 18–3).

Electrical signals sensed by demand pacemaker generators may originate not from the heart but from the environment (electrocautery, diathermy units, or microwave ovens) or the patient (muscle potentials). Such sensed signals may cause inhibition of inhibited units, leading to pauses in paced rhythm. Triggered generators are designed to emit output pulses upon sensing of signals, whatever their origin; thus, pauses in paced rhythm do not occur. Newer generator design and programmability have helped to reduce these "oversensing" problems.

The pacing function of a demand pulse generator cannot be evaluated if the patient's spontaneous rhythm exceeds the programmed rate of the generator. Application of a magnet over the generator converts it to an asynchronous mode of function, and capture (stimulation) of the atria or ventricles by

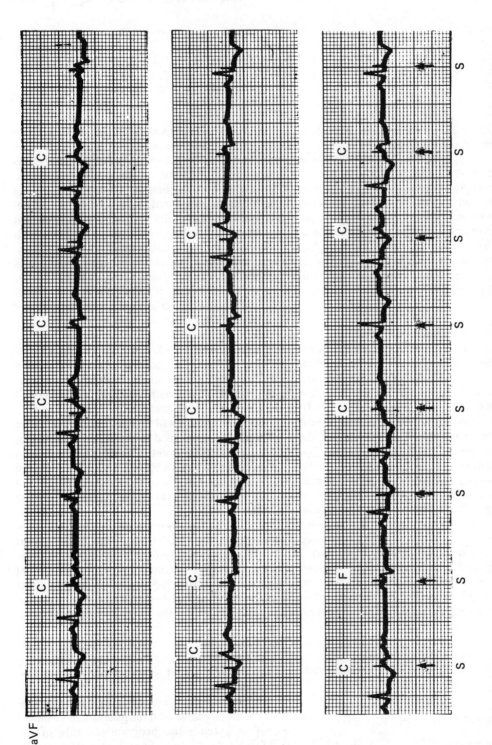

**Figure 18–1.** Asynchronous ventricular pacing (VOO) produced by placing a magnet over the implanted generator. Pacing stimuli (S) are delivered to the ventricle at the programmed rate of 65/min. Sensing of spontaneous QRS complexes does not occur, and the pacing stimuli are delivered at regular intervals. Pacing of the ventricles (C) occurs when ventricular tissue is not refractory. Several examples of sinus impulses conducted with delay or not conducted at all **(pseudo–AV block)** are present and are due to concealed retrograde conduction into the AV node by the paced ventricular complex. A fusion complex, in which the ventricles are depolarized from both the pacemaker and the sinus impulse, is seen in the bottom strip (third QRS complex, F).

Continuous recording

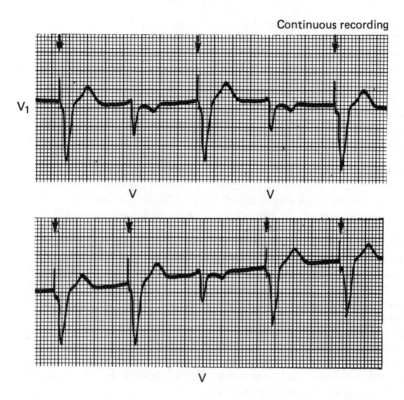

**Figure 18–2.** Ventricular-inhibited pacing (VVI). The generator has been programmed to pace at a rate of 75/min (interstimulus interval = 0.80 s), and output pulses are delivered 0.80 s after sensed spontaneous QRS complexes (V). When no spontaneous QRS complexes are sensed, ventricular pacing at the programmed rate occurs (arrows).

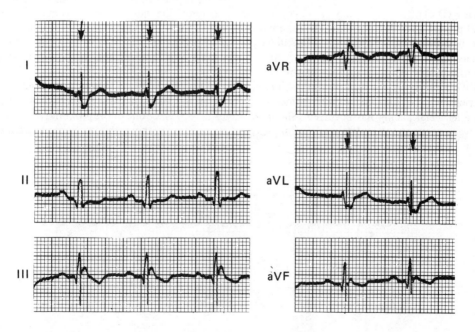

**Figure 18–3.** Triggered ventricular pacing (VVT). The QRS complexes are spontaneous and stimulated by the sinus P waves that precede them. Within each QRS complex, occurring about 40 ms after the onset of its inscription, is a pacing artifact (arrows), indicating that the complexes were sensed. The pacing artifacts do not contribute to ventricular activation. Triggered pacing might be confused with failure to sense unless the precise mode of function of the implanted generator is known.

the pacemaker can be confirmed, provided that the pacing stimuli fall outside the refractory period of the cardiac tissue (Fig 18–1). Conversely, if the patient is continually paced, the sensing function of the generator cannot be evaluated. Rate programming, in which the rate of the pulse generator is noninvasively and reversibly lowered, may allow a spontaneous cardiac rhythm to emerge, which should then be sensed.

### P-Synchronous Pacing (VAT & VDD)

P-synchronous pacing systems are dual-chamber systems, ie, electrodes are placed in both the atrium and the ventricle. When the atrial electrode senses an electrical signal, a ventricular pacing stimulus is delivered after a programmable **AV delay,** which corresponds roughly to the PR interval (Fig 18–4). Whereas earlier units (VAT) did not sense ventricular activity, thus resulting in the potential for competitive ventricular rhythms, newer devices (VDD) sense ventricular as well as atrial activity. Since sensing of atrial activity occurs with these devices, "tracking" of the atrial rhythm with a 1:1 AV conduction ratio occurs, allowing the patient to increase the ventricular paced rate along with the increase in the sinus rate. The generator is designed so as not to allow rapid ventricular paced rates to occur should the atrial rate become too fast. If no atrial activity is sensed, these pulse generators pace the ventricles on demand.

### AV Pacing (DVI)

DVI pacemaker generators have the capability of pacing both the atrium and the ventricle, but they sense only ventricular electrical activity. Since atrial sensing does not occur, the possibility of competitive atrial rhythms exists. With these units, the ventricles will be paced at the programmed AV interval after atrial pacing has occurred. Should a sinus P wave occur and stimulate a QRS complex,

some generators respond by inhibition of ventricular output and others by delivery of an output pulse at the end of the programmed AV delay, into the refractory period of ventricular tissue.

### Universal Pacing (DDD)

DDD generators are capable of sensing and pacing the atrium and of sensing and pacing the ventricle on demand (Fig 18–5). They thus approach the true physiology of normal AV conduction in many patients who require cardiac pacing. Problems associated with the use of DDD devices, as well as VDD devices, relate to their ability to sense retrograde atrial activity and stimulate the ventricles in response, thus creating an artificial extra-AV nodal bypass tract and causing a **pacemaker-mediated tachycardia.** Newer design features are expected to obviate these difficulties.

All dual-chamber devices depend upon a stable atrial rhythm for proper function. If the atrial rhythm is fibrillation, flutter, multifocal atrial tachycardia, or automatic tachycardia, these generators should not be implanted, and single-chamber ventricular-inhibited or ventricular-triggered devices should be implanted instead.

## UNIPOLAR & BIPOLAR PACING

Unipolar pacing systems have one electrode in the heart (the cathode) and the other electrode at the generator (the anode). The large distance between the cathode and anode in these systems results in large pacing artifacts whose direction in the frontal plane points toward the anode (generator) (Fig 18–6).

Bipolar pacing systems have both electrodes within the heart, usually 1–2 cm apart. Either the distal (tip) electrode or the proximal (ring) electrode may serve as the cathode. Because of the small

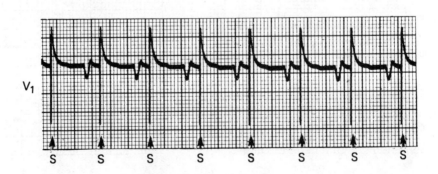

**Figure 18–4.** P-synchronous pacing (VDD). The atrial rhythm is sinus. After the (programmed) AV delay, a ventricular stimulus (S) is delivered. Thus, the ventricular paced rate is the same as the sinus rate. Should the atrial rate become very rapid, specific pacemaker design features disallow 1:1 AV pacing in order to protect the ventricles from a rapid paced rate. If spontaneous P wave activity does not occur, the generator paces the ventricles on demand at its programmed rate.

Continuous recording

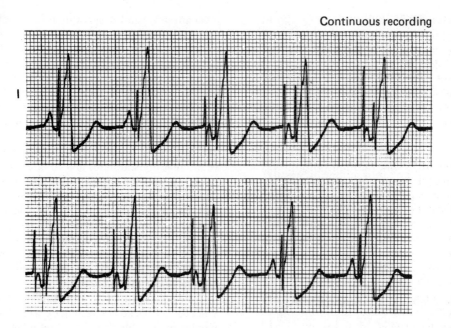

**Figure 18–5.** Atrial and ventricular pacing in a DDD pacing system. The first two P waves are sinus and inhibit the atrial pacing output circuit. The atrial rate then slows slightly, and the remaining P waves are paced at the programmed rate of 72/min. All QRS complexes are paced, since no spontaneous QRS complexes occur within the programmed AV interval of 0.14 s. Had a spontaneous QRS complex been stimulated by either a sinus or paced P wave, the ventricular output would have been inhibited.

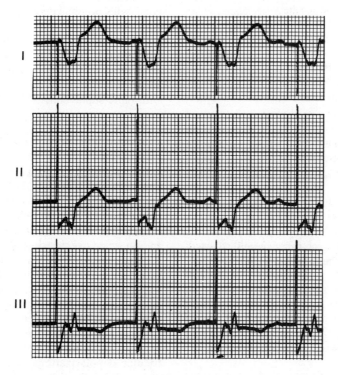

**Figure 18–6.** Unipolar ventricular pacing system implanted on the left ventricular epicardial surface during cardiac surgery. The large amplitude of the pacing stimuli indicates that this is a unipolar system. The axis of the pacing artifacts is inferiorly directed, indicating that the generator lies inferior to the heart (it was in the upper abdominal wall). The paced QRS complexes have a right bundle branch block pattern, consistent with left ventricular activation occurring earlier than right ventricular activation.

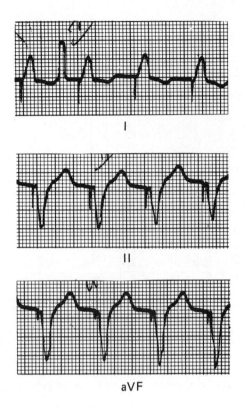

I

II

aVF

**Figure 18–7.** Bipolar ventricular pacing. The pacing artifacts have a small amplitude, indicating a small interelectrode distance. They are negatively directed in leads II and III, reflecting an inferior to superior direction of current flow. Thus, the distal (tip) electrode has been made negative and the proximal (ring) electrode has been made positive, with current traveling from tip to ring.

interelectrode distance, the pacing artifact is small and its direction in the frontal plane reflects the direction of current flow (Fig 18–7).

## ELECTROCARDIOGRAPHIC PATTERNS OF PACED COMPLEXES

The configurations of paced complexes will depend upon how the myocardium is depolarized. Paced atrial complexes will reflect the sequence of atrial activation initiated by the pacing impulse and thus, in part, the site of the pacing electrode. Since the atrial electrodes may be located in the atrial appendage or screwed into any portion of atrial tissue, paced P waves will have variable contours (Figs 18–5 and 18–8).

Pacing from the right ventricular endocardial or epicardial apical area will produce QRS complexes that have a left bundle branch block configuration (since the right ventricular myocardium is depolarized in advance of the left ventricular

myocardium), and a superior mean frontal plane axis (since the apex of the heart is depolarized before the base) (Fig 18–9A and 18–9B). Paced QRS complexes usually have a duration of 0.12–0.18 s; if they are substantially longer, intrinsic myocardial disease should be suspected.

Pacing from the right ventricular outflow tract results in QRS complexes that have a left bundle branch block pattern (since the right ventricular myocardium is depolarized in advance of the left ventricular myocardium) and an inferiorly directed mean frontal plane axis (since the base of the heart is depolarized before the apex) (Fig 18–9C). Occasionally, pacing from high on the interventricular septum can result in paced QRS complexes that show an indeterminate conduction delay pattern or even a narrow complex, reflecting activation of both the right and left sides of the interventricular septum nearly simultaneously.

Pacing from the left ventricular epicardium will produce paced QRS complexes that have a right bundle branch block pattern, reflecting left ventricular myocardial activation in advance of right ventricular activation (Fig 18–6). The mean frontal plane QRS axis will depend upon the location of the epicardial electrodes relative to each other (bipolar system) or to the pulse generator (unipolar system).

Spontaneous QRS complexes occurring in patients with pacemakers often show T wave inversion. Although the cause of the T wave inversion is not understood, it should not be interpreted to indicate myocardial disease. Similar T wave abnormalities may be seen in patients with intermittent intraventricular conduction delays and in patients with rapid supraventricular tachyarrhythmias.

## PACEMAKER MALFUNCTION

The general categories of pacemaker malfunction are failure to sense and failure to capture. Sensing of unwanted electrical signals (such as T waves, myopotentials, and environmental signals such as electrocautery) does *not* represent failure to sense and is termed **oversensing.** Programming the pulse generator to "see" electrical signals of larger magnitude will often solve the problem. Conversely, **undersensing** of electrical signals due to poor signal quality may represent not sensing failure but rather the suboptimal nature of the signal itself. Undersensed QRS complexes are not rare and tend to originate in ventricular tissue (premature ventricular depolarizations) or occur during acute myocardial infarction or because of drug toxicity and electrolyte imbalance (Fig 18–10).

Failure to sense spontaneous complexes results in the delivery of a pacing stimulus earlier than expected (Fig 18–10). This may cause competitive

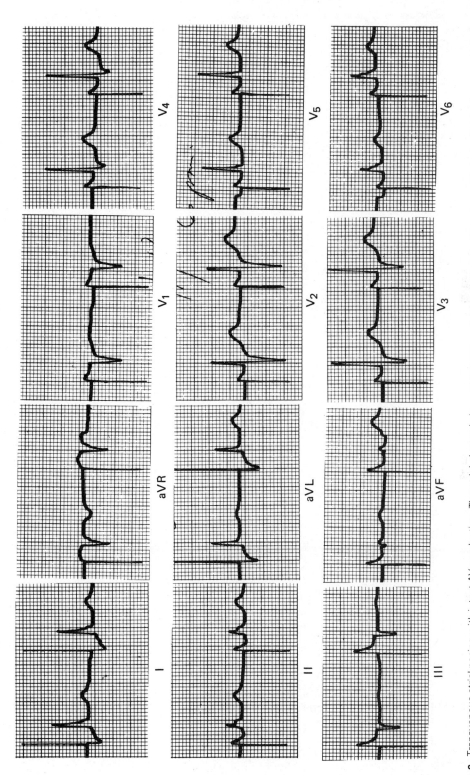

**Figure 18—8.** Transvenous atrial pacing with intact AV conduction. The atrial electrode is unipolar, accounting for the large pacing artifacts. The large artifact and its associated decay curve often obscure the contour of the paced P waves. In this tracing, the paced P waves are upright in II, III, and aVF and negative in I and aVL. Since the P wave vector is directed inferiorly and rightward, the atrial electrode is located in the high right atrium.

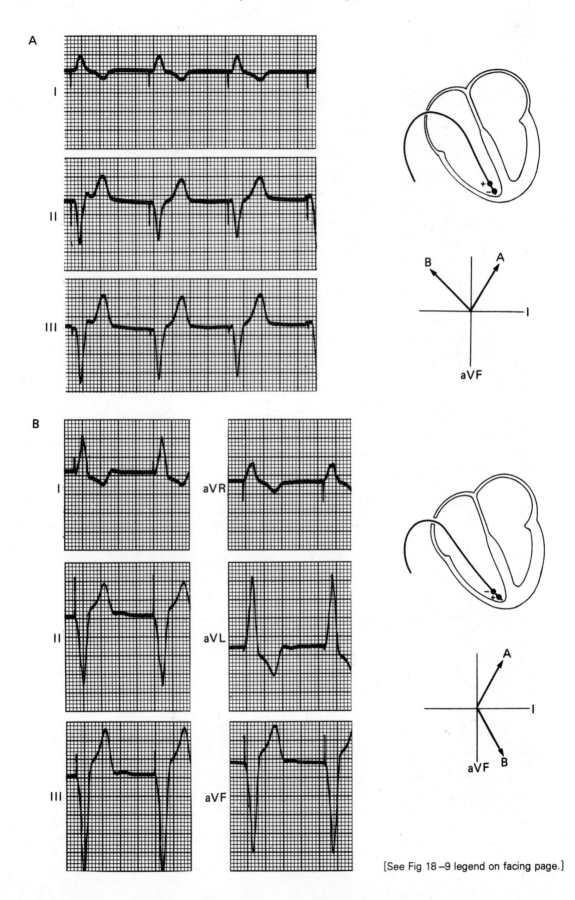

[See Fig 18–9 legend on facing page.]

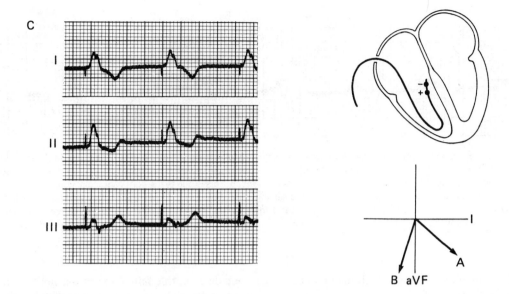

**Figure 18–9.** Diagrammatic illustrations of bipolar pacing systems. *A:* The pacing catheter is located in the right ventricular apical area. The distal (tip) electrode is the cathode and the proximal (ring) electrode is the anode. The pacing artifact is small because of the small interelectrode distance. Since current flows from cathode to anode, the pacing artifact axis is oriented rightward and superiorly (arrow B), producing small negative deflections in I, II, and III. The myocardium is depolarized leftward and superiorly (arrow A), resulting in upright QRS complexes in lead I and negative QRS complexes in II and III. *B:* The distal (tip) electrode is the anode and the proximal (ring) electrode is the cathode. The pacing artifact is oriented leftward and inferiorly (arrow B), resulting in upright deflections in II, III, and aVF. The myocardium is depolarized leftward and superiorly (arrow A), resulting in upright QRS complexes in leads I and aVL and negative complexes in II, III, and aVF. *C:* The pacing catheter is located in the outflow tract of the right ventricle. Current flows from cathode to anode (tip to ring), and thus the pacing artifacts are directed inferiorly, resulting in upright deflections in II and III. Since current is also flowing from left to right in this diagram, the pacing artifact is negative in lead I. The myocardium is depolarized from base to apex, resulting in upright QRS complexes in II and III.

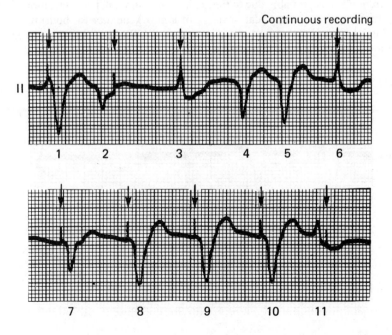

**Figure 18–10.** Intermittent "failure" to sense. Pacing stimuli are delivered earlier than expected (QRS complexes 2, 3, 6, and 11), indicating failure to sense those complexes, which is probably due to their poor signal quality. The delivery of pacing stimuli in the ventricular vulnerable period could result in repetitive ventricular rhythms.

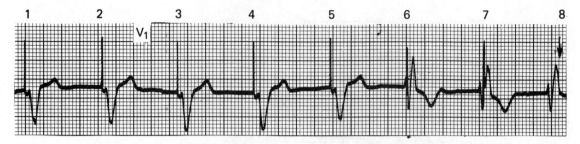

**Figure 18–11.** Transvenous right ventricular **demand pacing** system with electrode catheter located in the right ventricular apex. QRS complexes 6, 7, and 8 are spontaneous and show a right bundle branch block configuration. The first 2 of these have pacing artifacts within them, indicating that they were not sensed. This is due to the right ventricular conduction delay, with consequent late arrival at the electrode of the ventricular activation wave front. This does not represent sensing failure. As the differential diagnosis of this rhythm strip includes **triggered pacing** with episodic failure to sense those QRS complexes not containing a pacing artifact within them, knowledge of the mode of function of the implanted device is mandatory.

atrial or ventricular rhythms, which may on occasion be life-threatening.

Occasionally, in patients with transvenous right ventricular VVI pacing systems, pacing artifacts occur within spontaneous QRS complexes having a right bundle branch block configuration (Fig 18–11). Failure to sense QRS complexes having a right bundle branch block pattern indicates that, because of the delay in conduction in the right bundle branch, the wave of ventricular depolarization did not reach the area of the pacing catheter in the right ventricular apex before the pacing stimulus was due to arrive. This phenomenon may also be observed in patients with inferior and right ventricular myocardial infarction and is probably due to the conduction delay resulting from ventricular scarring. Because failure to "see" the wave front of ventricular activation is due to intrinsic conduction

system disease, true failure to sense is not present. The same principles apply to patients with left ventricular epicardial electrodes who have underlying left bundle branch block.

Failure to pace is present when pacing stimuli do not depolarize myocardium (Fig 18–12). This may result from poor electrode position, from pulse generator output reduction (battery end-of-life), or from an increase in myocardial stimulation threshold due to acute myocardial infarction, drug toxicity, electrolyte imbalance, cardiopulmonary resuscitation, or fibrosis at the pacing catheter tip. Pacing failure can be managed acutely by noninvasive programming of the energy output of the generator to its maximum, but lead repositioning or implantation of a new generator (or both) may be required, depending upon the underlying problem.

Continuous recording

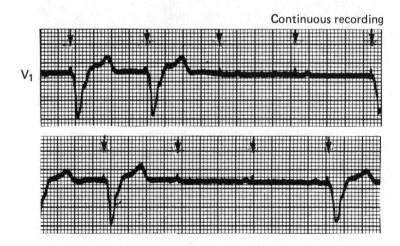

**Figure 18–12.** Intermittent failure to capture. Pacing artifacts are indicated by the arrows. Long pauses in paced rhythm, during which pacing artifacts occur but do not stimulate QRS complexes, indicate failure to pace. The problem could be due to generator failure or an increase in the myocardial stimulation threshold.

# TEST TRACINGS

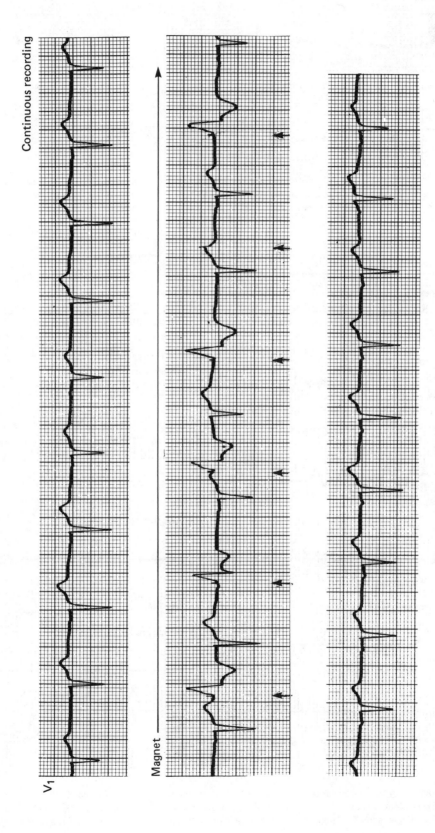

**Figure 18–T1.** Ventricular-inhibited (VVI) pacing. The upper and lower strips show sinus rhythm with normal AV conduction. During application of a magnet (middle strip), the pulse generator is converted to an asynchronous (VOO) mode of function (rate, 50/min), in which sensing does not occur. Capture of the ventricles by the pacemaker occurs when ventricular tissue is nonrefractory. It is important to note that unless it is known that the magnet had been applied, sensing malfunction could have been diagnosed.

Continuous recording

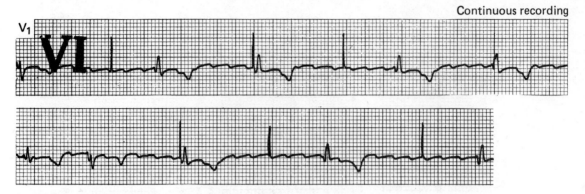

**Figure 18–T2.** Failure to pace. This VVI pacemaker was set to pace at 60/min. All QRS complexes are spontaneous; those that fall after delivery of a pacer output pulse and therefore within the refractory period of the pacemaker generator are appropriately not sensed. Failure to pace is diagnosed by the presence of pacing artifacts that do not stimulate QRS complexes.

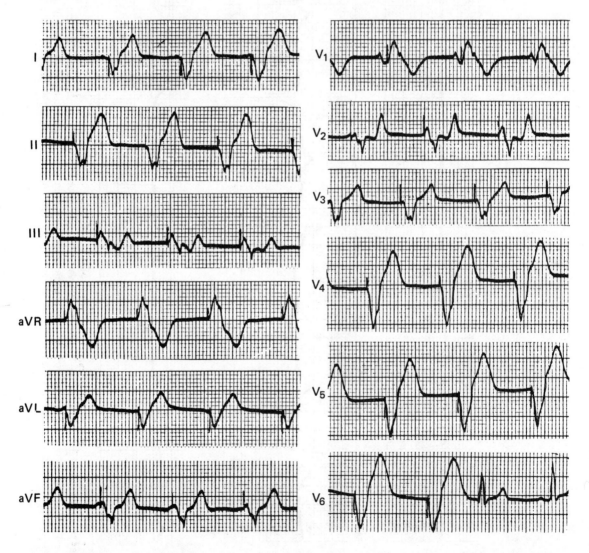

**Figure 18–T3.** Bipolar ventricular pacemaker located on the left ventricular epicardial surface. The QRS complexes have a right bundle branch block configuration, indicating a left ventricular location of the electrodes. The mean frontal plane axis of the paced QRS complexes will be determined by the location of the electrodes and by their respective polarities.

## PERICARDITIS

The earliest electrocardiographic evidence of pericarditis is ST segment elevation in those leads overlying the involved area, reflecting epicardial injury current. Thus, the ST segment elevation may be diffuse or localized. The ST segment elevation is typically concave upward, in contrast to that of acute myocardial infarction, which is convex upward (Fig 19–1). Lead aVR or $V_1$ (or both) may show (reciprocal) ST segment depression (Fig 19–1). After days or weeks, depending upon the clinical course of the pericarditis, the ST segments become isoelectric and the T waves inverted (Figs 19–1, 19–2, and 19–3). Occasionally, the ST elevation resolves without T wave inversion, or T wave inversion may occur and persist for months. Abnormal Q waves are not present in pericarditis.

In pericarditis with effusion, *serial* ECGs may show a decrease in voltage of P waves and QRS complexes. **Electrical alternans** may occur (Figs 19–4 and 19–5). Electrical alternans, in which the height of the complexes alternates, can involve the QRS complexes, P waves, T waves, U waves, and even the ST segments. Its genesis is poorly understood. Electrical alternans is seen in severe heart disease due to any cause as well as in pericardial effusion and is therefore not specific for this diagnosis. Electrical alternans should not be confused with **mechanical (pulsus) alternans,** in which alternating ventricular contractions produce blood pressures of alternating magnitude.

PR segment depression is commonly seen in pericarditis (Fig 19–1). This represents prominence of the atrial repolarization wave and may reflect atrial involvement in the pericardial process. Because PR segment depression is also seen in atrial infarction and during exercise, it is not specific for the diagnosis of pericarditis.

## MYOCARDITIS

Any acute or chronic disease can involve the myocardium and thereby result in electrocardio-

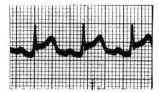

Concave ST elevation
in pericarditis

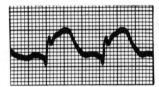

Convex ST elevation
in infarction

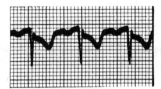

Cavity complex;
pericarditis

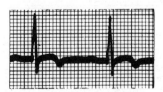

Late pattern; pericarditis

**Figure 19–1.** Electrocardiographic patterns in pericarditis and myocardial infarction.

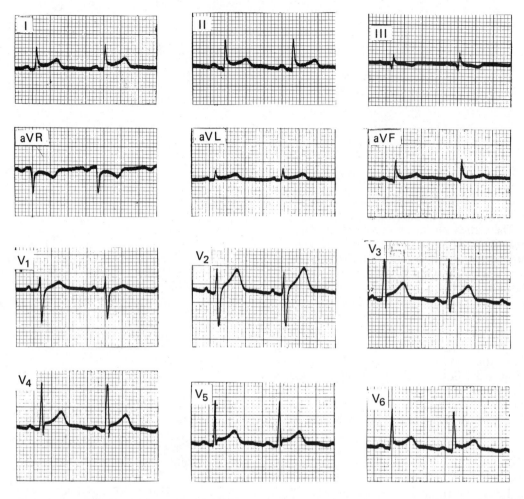

**Figure 19–2.** Acute pericarditis. ST segment elevation with concave upward curvature is seen in leads I, II, aVL, and $V_{2-6}$. Reciprocal ST segment depression is seen in lead aVR.

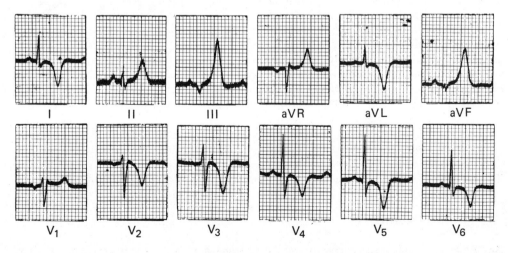

**Figure 19–3.** Pericarditis (late pattern). Deep, symmetrically inverted T waves in I, aVL, and $V_{2-6}$. The marked T wave abnormalities, unusual in pericarditis, may indicate concomitant myocarditis.

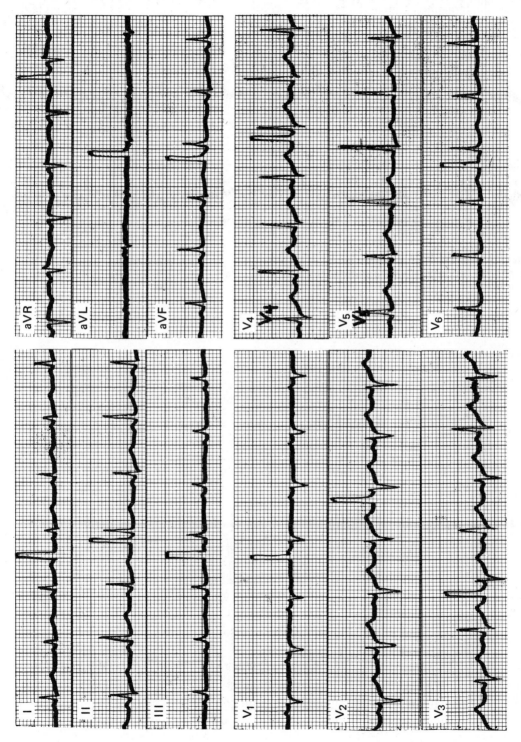

**Figure 19–4.** Electrical alternans. The rhythm is sinus. The QRS morphology (and polarity in some leads) alternates in an absolutely regular fashion.

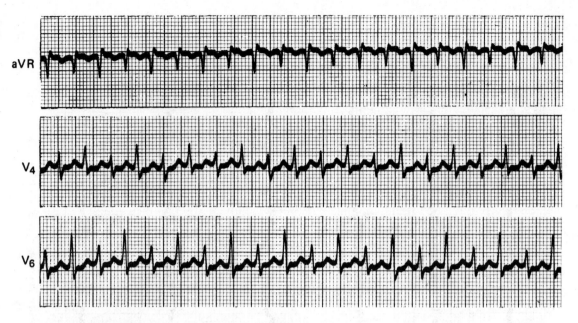

**Figure 19–5.** Apparent electrical alternans. The rhythm is a reentry supraventricular tachycardia with a rate of 200/min. The alternation of the QRS amplitude in the presence of reentry tachycardia does not represent electrical alternans but rather reflects antegrade conduction to the ventricles over 2 pathways in alternating fashion.

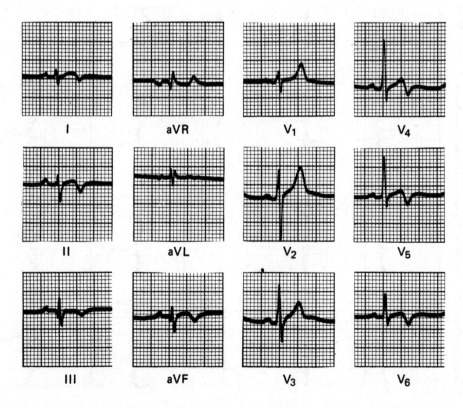

**Figure 19–6.** Abnormal ECG with nondiagnostic ST–T wave abnormalities. The T waves are deeply and symmetrically inverted in I, II, III, and $V_{4–6}$, suggesting a diffuse myocardial process. The clinical diagnosis was acute viral myocarditis in a 22-year-old man.

graphic abnormalities that are not specific for a particular diagnosis. These abnormalities include the following: (1) prolongation of the PR interval; (2) arrhythmias; (3) ST segment abnormalities; (4) isolated T wave abnormalities; (5) prolongation of the QT interval; and (6) changes in the QRS configuration, which may mimic myocardial infarction (Fig 19–6). Since the electrocardiographic changes are nondiagnostic, close clinical correlation is mandatory.

## HYPERTHYROIDISM

The usual electrocardiographic findings in hyperthyroidism are sinus tachycardia and nonspecific ST and T wave abnormalities (Fig 19–7). Atrial fibrillation with a very rapid ventricular rate (due to enhanced AV nodal conduction of the fibrillatory impulses) may also be seen. The abnormalities are

expected to resolve with treatment of the hyperthyroidism, but normalization of the ECG may take weeks to months.

## MYXEDEMA

Electrocardiographic features suggesting myxedema include sinus bradycardia, prolongation of the PR interval, low QRS and P wave voltages, and flat T waves (Fig 19–8). As with hyperthyroidism, these abnormalities regress with treatment of the myxedema, but that may take weeks to months.

## TRAUMATIC HEART DISEASE

Trauma to the heart can produce coronary artery laceration, coronary artery thrombosis, and

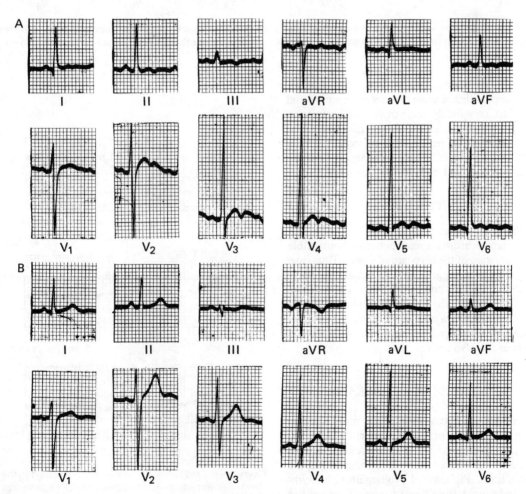

**Figure 19–7.** Hyperthyroidism. *A:* Taken prior to therapy for hyperthyroidism. Rate = 110/min. The T waves are inverted in I, II, III, aVF, and $V_6$, flat in aVL, and diphasic in $V_{2-5}$. These changes are nonspecific. $RV_5 + SV_1 = 40$ mm. Ordinarily, this would be suggestive of left ventricular hypertrophy, but these voltage criteria are invalid in the presence of hyperthyroidism. *B:* ECG recorded when patient was euthyroid.

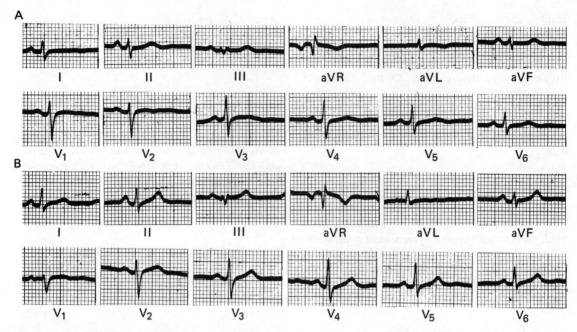

**Figure 19–8.** Myxedema. *A:* The QRS complexes are of low voltage and the T waves of low amplitude in all leads. *B:* Three weeks after thyroid therapy: The T waves are now of normal amplitude, and there is a slight increase in the QRS voltage.

myocardial contusion. The ECG may therefore reflect abnormalities of acute myocardial necrosis and may mimic completely acute myocardial infarction due to coronary artery disease. Electrocardiographic patterns of pericarditis are common (Fig 19–9). Supraventricular and ventricular arrhythmias may occur and may be life-threatening.

## TUMOR

Primary or metastatic tumor of the heart produces electrocardiographic patterns compatible with infiltration of the myocardial tissue. Thus, low voltage, q waves suggesting myocardial infarction, and intraventricular conduction delays may all be seen (Fig 19–10). The low voltage may be due to replacement of the myocardium by tumor tissue or to associated malignant pericardial effusion. Arrhythmias are also seen.

## NEUROMUSCULAR DISEASES

Friedreich's ataxia, progressive muscular dystrophy (Duchenne or pseudohypertrophic), and myotonia dystrophica are neuromuscular diseases commonly associated with electrocardiographic abnormalities. PR interval prolongation, arrhythmias, and nonspecific ST and T wave abnormalities are the changes most commonly observed, but hypertrophy patterns and deviation of the mean frontal plane QRS axis also occur.

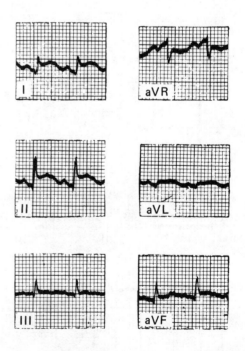

**Figure 19–9.** Cardiac trauma due to gunshot wound to the chest. ST segment elevation is present in all leads except aVR, which shows ST depression. PR segment depression is seen in I, II, and aVF. These diffuse changes could reflect pericarditis and myocarditis or myocardial necrosis; serial ECGs are required for correct interpretation.

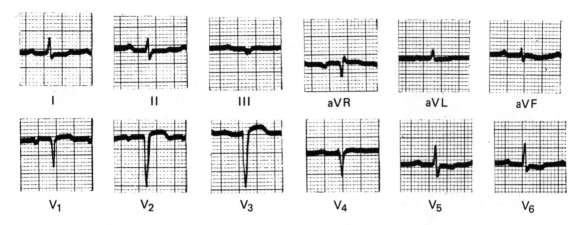

**Figure 19–10.** Metastatic bronchogenic carcinoma involving the heart. The QRS complexes have low voltage in the limb leads. QS complexes are present in V₁₋₂, and ST segment elevation is seen in V₂₋₃. Although these findings might suggest anterior wall myocardial infarction due to coronary disease, in this case they are due to replacement of the myocardium by tumor tissue. The ECG records the electrically "dead" or "silent" area of tissue but cannot, of course, distinguish its cause.

## HYPOTHERMIA

The electrocardiographic manifestations of hypothermia include sinus bradycardia (often extreme), atrial fibrillation, escape rhythms, prolongation of the QT interval, and Osborne ("J") waves. The J waves are waves inscribed at the terminal portion of the QRS complexes, before the ST segment and T wave (Fig 19–11). They should not be mistaken for portions of QRS complexes or for ST segment elevation. J waves, atrial fibrillation, and ventricular fibrillation reflect severe hypothermia (25° C or less).

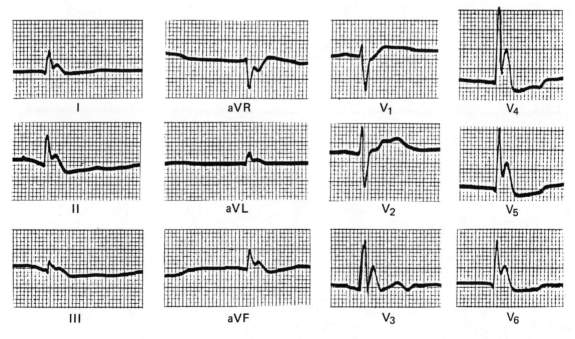

**Figure 19–11.** Hypothermia. The ventricular rate is 50/min. Atrial activity is not seen. The QRS complexes are narrow and are deformed at their terminal portions by a slurred wave occurring prior to the inscription of the ST–T waves; this is the J wave. The QT interval is prolonged. (Courtesy of R Brindis, MD.)

# Index